AF867463

Sustainable Health and the COVID-19 Crisis

Interdisciplinary Perspectives

This edited collection offers interdisciplinary perspectives on some of the key health challenges faced by individuals, communities, and governments during the COVID-19 pandemic. Taking the Danish context as a starting point, it extrapolates to discuss the international relevance of a range of issues.

The book contains four parts:

- Part 1 looks at the societal reactions to COVID-19, discussing issues around health communication, legitimacy, ethics, and bio-politics.
- Part 2 approaches the health and well-being of specific groups during the crisis.
- Part 3 assesses how the crisis stimulated sustainable solutions to key problems, from digital methods for the delivery of health care, to changes to the food supply chain.
- Part 4 looks broadly at how historical developments in the study of epidemiology and current scientific perspectives enable the understanding and, to some extent, management of the COVID-19 pandemic.

With contributions from scholars across the social sciences, health sciences, and humanities, each chapter provides not only insight into a particular issue, but also the theories and scientific methods applied to understand and overcome the COVID-19 crisis. It will be important reading for both scholars and policy makers, informing an appropriate response to future health crises.

Nicole Thualagant is an associate professor and head of Study in Critical Health Studies at the University of Roskilde. She is also a member of the scientific committee in the Nordic Health Promotion Research Network meeting twice a year at WHO in Copenhagen. As a sociologist, her interest is in health policies, more especially how health policies interfere with more intimate spheres of social life in contemporary welfare societies.

Pelle Korsbæk Sørensen is a lecturer in nursing at the Research & Development Unit at University College Absalon, Denmark. He is the former chairperson of the Nordic Sociological Association (2016–2018). He makes use of different methodological approaches, and he teaches research design and mixed methods. His interest is in sociology of health and his main areas of research are moral and ethical distress and psychosocial working environment among health professionals.

Troels Sune Mønsted is an associate professor in digitalization of healthcare at the Department of Informatics, University of Oslo. He is a member of the board of the Danish Society for Digital Health and is affiliated to the HISP Centre (Health Information Systems Program), Oslo. In his research, he combines qualitative methods and action research in investigating design and use of patient-centred technologies and information infrastructures in healthcare.

Sustainable Health and the COVID-19 Crisis

Interdisciplinary Perspectives

Edited by Nicole Thualagant,
Pelle Korsbæk Sørensen, and
Troels Sune Mønsted

Routledge
Taylor & Francis Group
LONDON AND NEW YORK

First published 2024
by Routledge
4 Park Square, Milton Park, Abingdon, Oxon OX14 4RN

and by Routledge
605 Third Avenue, New York, NY 10158

Routledge is an imprint of the Taylor & Francis Group, an informa business

© 2024 selection and editorial matter, Nicole Thualagant and Pelle Korsbæk Sørensen and Troels Sune Mønsted; individual chapters, the contributors

The right of Nicole Thualagant and Pelle Korsbæk Sørensen and Troels Sune Mønsted to be identified as the authors of the editorial material, and of the authors for their individual chapters, has been asserted in accordance with sections 77 and 78 of the Copyright, Designs and Patents Act 1988.

All rights reserved. No part of this book may be reprinted or reproduced or utilised in any form or by any electronic, mechanical, or other means, now known or hereafter invented, including photocopying and recording, or in any information storage or retrieval system, without permission in writing from the publishers.

Trademark notice: Product or corporate names may be trademarks or registered trademarks, and are used only for identification and explanation without intent to infringe.

British Library Cataloguing-in-Publication Data
A catalogue record for this book is available from the British Library

ISBN: 978-1-032-25778-5 (hbk)
ISBN: 978-1-032-57980-1 (pbk)
ISBN: 978-1-003-44191-5 (ebk)

DOI: 10.4324/9781003441915

Typeset in Sabon
by MPS Limited, Dehradun

Contents

Preface

This edited collection is the product of extensive interdisciplinary cooperation between researchers interested in the questions of sustainability, health, and welfare. More precisely, it is a product embedded in the 'Health and Welfare' research network, in which colleagues from four departments of Roskilde University, Denmark, met regularly to discuss research related to issues of health and welfare. In 2019, scholars from the Research Centre in Health Promotion took the initiative to gather researchers from all four departments (People and Technology, Social Sciences and Business, Science and Environment, Communication and Arts) to create an open space and platform for interdisciplinary exchange and development of research on the interconnectedness between sustainability, health, and welfare. This network soon became a venue for shared research interests and ambitions for a collective work. While discussions were being fuelled on how we, as a large research community, could develop our research and explore it across disciplinary boundaries, the first tentative warnings and concerns regarding a new virus presented themselves. The COVID-19 pandemic started. The COVID-19 context then became a central health crisis to explore and joint efforts were made to create a book proposal. Through regular meetings (first on campus, but later online as the pandemic spread), the researchers who started out as coordinators of the interdisciplinary network also became editors of this collection.

Although Denmark is the point of reference in the analyses, the scope is international. Many of the chapters cross boundaries in scientific terms and borders in terms of nation-states, showing the interdependent and globalised nature of scientific disciplines and politics. In a pandemic, no problem stays local for long.

Many of the authors are based at Roskilde University in Denmark, although authors from other educational institutions joined the process and some ventured to other institutions, nationally and internationally. It is our sincere hope that this edited collection will be read across boundaries and borders, and that scholars, students, and policymakers will draw inspiration from this interdisciplinary work in order to facilitate reactions to future crises.

Interdisciplinarity not only created a suitable opportunity for developing a book proposal on COVID-19 as a crisis involving both health and welfare, it also nourished the making of the project of an edited collection and contributed later in the peer-review process. Not only is this edited collection the fruit of interdisciplinary joint efforts, each contribution is deeply anchored in an interdisciplinary ontology and has been discussed and approved through a double-blinded review process offering different lenses on the contribution.

As editors, it is high time for us to thank the external reviewers who exemplarily read each contribution on its own terms, the members of the network who nourished the many discussions and contributed to the edited collection, Roskilde University for hosting us and providing funding, Routledge for enabling us to fulfil this project, and our proofreader who provided coherency between the texts.

Tables

Figures

1 Introductory thoughts on exploring the COVID-19 crisis through interdisciplinary lenses

Nicole Thualagant, Troels Mønsted, and Pelle Korsbæk Sørensen

During the course of history, global crises have had a significant impact on societies, not only by disrupting everyday life on a short-term basis and shaping societal development in general, but also by influencing what we perceive to be a sustainable future. In different ways, these crises, such as the financial or climate crisis, encourage nation-states to devise immediate political and social responses as well as engaging various scientific disciplines to mitigate the highly complex challenges involved. Global crises have, beyond their obvious harmful effects, also propelled developments in, e.g., technology, medicine, economics, and politics, and hence had a significant influence on the trajectories leading to our current societies. The purpose of this book is to take stock of how the COVID-19 pandemic influenced both the short-term sustainability perspective and the long-term perspective of health care provision in a welfare state, in this case Denmark.

This edited collection focuses on health from a broad perspective, in the sense that health is much more than just the absence of disease or infirmity. In fact, health is deeply interconnected with sustainability and has become one of the most central issues of contemporary society. Individual health is linked directly to the progress and prosperity of welfare states, as healthy populations are a resource and less of a drain on public budgets. Following this line of thought, the World Health Organization (WHO) has for several decades advised countries to implement a whole-of-government and whole-of-society approach to equitable improvement in health, i.e., a policy framework and strategy supporting health promotion on many levels of government and governance.

This edited collection investigates the consequences of and responses to a global crisis in a welfare state with a specific focus on the provision and maintenance of health. An obvious objective for a 21st century universal welfare state is to provide health care in accordance with global standards of sustainability (Jelsøe et al., 2018). In this light, health encompasses social, environmental, and economic dimensions and is thus intertwined with a general focus on sustainability. From an ecological perspective, health is both a collective and individual concern that is vital for the sustainability of society in a welfare state (Richard et al., 2011). Welfare states are in a

DOI: 10.4324/9781003441915-1

constant state of development to match the provision of common goods to the needs of the citizens and to changing conditions in global society, and thus face a range of transitions, changes, and transformations. These are often linked directly to different crises affecting legislation, norms, and the everyday life of citizens. In addition, scientific developments follow in the wake of a deep-rooted crisis. COVID-19 is an example of such a groundbreaking crisis that put the welfare state to the test.

The challenges for health care systems resulting from the COVID-19 pandemic were highly complex, cross-cutting and *wicked* (Rittel & Webber, 1973) in the sense that the question of how to address the health risks for the population while maintaining a functional society was difficult to find answers to and laden with contradictory and changing requirements and conditions. Further, COVID-19 produced cascading challenges, where solutions to one problem resulted in the emergence of other problems. More specifically, COVID-19 accelerated the development of global vaccination and disease tracking programmes, but also forced societies to find ways to adapt to and cope with not only the disease itself but also its complex ramifications at the individual and societal levels, such as social and working life, production and the economy, and the delivery of public services. A range of emergent problems needed urgent solutions, such as how to take care of vulnerable people or population groups that were particularly affected by the crisis, communicate the necessity of new legislation, ensure financial stability, and reorganise industries. As a result, the societal challenges that emerged during COVID-19 were not easily solved or understood within the confines of traditional scientific disciplines. For the same reason, the pandemic proved to be an opportune moment for interdisciplinary research to develop nuanced understandings of the challenges that emerge during times of crisis, the individual and societal consequences and their interconnectedness, and responses to these consequences. In this logic, COVID-19 caused many crises in one crisis: it was primarily a health crisis, yet it also became a financial crisis, a social crisis and a mental health crisis. In other words, it became a crisis that was central to the research questions and research fields we present in this edited collection.

This collection will mainly deal with Denmark as an example or case of a welfare state, although the issues raised via this lens have an inherent global character. One common point of reference provides the collection of chapters with a path of stepping stones to follow for the reader. As the following chapters will show, taking a small country as our basis can highlight tendencies shared across the globe; for example, care of elderly or disabled people, discussions about wearing face masks in public, or the justification for calling for a lockdown of society have been topics to address in all countries during COVID-19. The pandemic showed that individual countries could impose travel restrictions, yet the problems to be solved were transnational, and just like the disease they could not be contained.

The study of COVID-19 as a real-world problem

The pandemic situation that originated in late 2019 and challenged welfare states globally was yet another crisis among other global crises highlighting the severe vulnerability of our very existence. What characterises these global crises is the complexity of real-world problems. COVID-19 was not just a matter of another virus causing ill health and sometimes death. COVID-19 came unexpectedly with major uncertainty as to the nature of the virus and was rapidly identified as an important challenge to health and in the longer-term economic and social stability.

Complex real-world problems highlight the relevance of interdisciplinary approaches and analyses. Unidisciplinary approaches can rarely embrace their complexities. This book brings together more than 25 authors from diverse research fields with a common aim to analyse the problem of COVID-19 in a welfare state, not only in terms of its implications for health maintenance and promotion in contemporary society, but also its implications for current research fields. The focus in this edited collection is the Danish context, with its provision of the common good of health in a welfare society in a time of crisis. Nonetheless, the analyses presented are of relevance in enhancing our understanding of the recent health crisis, which, as argued in the epilogue, also applies to the context of other societies.

The contributions of this edited collection are knowledge produced based on research conducted within an academic tradition of problem orientation. As a key aspect of this approach to research that is deeply rooted in real-world problems and suggests solutions to these, the contributions all engage with interdisciplinarity and problem orientation. Problem-oriented research often stands in contrast to basic research because of its approach and objective. Contrary to basic research aiming at new general scientific findings, problem-oriented research aims at exploring how general knowledge can be applied to real-world problems that cannot be solved in a unidisciplinary manner (Conrad, 2002; Kueffer et al., 2012).

Problem-oriented research can be embedded in different ontological traditions and theoretical understandings. However, what generally characterises problem-oriented research is the recognition that real-world problems are often complex, heterogeneous, and perceived differently by actors in the problem domain. Finding the root of the problem is therefore rarely a linear process, but requires persistent exploration through different perspectives. In this spirit, the objective of this edited collection is to present the reader with a range of interdisciplinary analyses to enable a deeper understanding of the complexities of the societal challenges faced during COVID-19 (Mol & Law, 2002).

Why interdisciplinary lenses?

Categories such as 'multi-, inter-, cross-, pluri-, and trans-' disciplinarity have been highlighted as the grand solution to complex real-world problems in recent decades and emphasised the practical relevance of science. Cross-disciplinarity was pointed out as a way to achieve more nuanced understandings and analyses of complexity in the aftermath of the Second World War and in the emerging focus on global crises such as the climate crisis. In 1970, the Organisation for Economic Co-operation and Development (OECD) placed high hopes on interdisciplinarity; it was presented as the solution to the social demands of the time. Moreover, universities were encouraged to develop more radical methods of teaching and conducting research that crossed disciplinary boundaries (OECD, 1972). Despite the original enthusiasm, OECD declared in a publication from 1985 that the invitation to interdisciplinarity had not been accepted, since traditional disciplines even seemed strengthened in many traditional universities. However, the idea of making interdisciplinarity more of a question of ontology than of epistemology has inspired numerous researchers and research institutions. Here, the focus on letting pressing real-world problems define what and how interdisciplinarity can be relevant has inspired many researchers and the so-called reform universities that emerged in the late 1960s and early 1970s. In these scientific milieus, the focus is not on interdisciplinarity as a methodological question, but on interdisciplinarity as leading to ontological change. We would argue that the intention of letting real-world problems define the relevance of interdisciplinarity is preventing us from understanding interdisciplinarity as a synthesis or integration of disciplines. Neither should we understand interdisciplinarity as a 'subordination-service model' (Barry et al., 2008), where some disciplines are in the service of higher-ranked disciplines. Interdisciplinarity as problem-solving permits us to encourage more nuanced analyses of complex world challenges. However, this approach to interdisciplinarity demands a reflective approach to what constitutes 'a problem'. Inspired by Barry et al., we would argue that problems should be understood '(…) as constituted as interdisciplinary problems relationally through dialogue or dissatisfaction with the problematics proffered by existing disciplines and institutions' (2008, p. 30).

The COVID-19 crisis gave rise to new reflections on the notion of interdisciplinarity. This edited collection offers an insight into how interdisciplinary and problem-oriented research can advance an understanding of the challenges posed by a crisis in a welfare state. Fundamental to the book is a scientific dialogue based on interdisciplinary approaches to health in welfare states through the lenses of various research fields in the social sciences, humanities, and natural sciences. The strength of an interdisciplinary approach to a societal crisis in the form of a problem-oriented approach to knowledge production has previously been emphasised, and the relevance of interdisciplinarity did not diminish in the complexity of the COVID-19 situation. Many of the analyses in this collection are inherently interdisciplinary. This lies in the heart of critical and problem-based research. The researchers draw on more than one discipline to answer their research questions. As a result, they present multifaceted analyses and present solutions that reject reductionism. This is in line with the notion that it never should be a conclusion that a phenomenon is complex (Mol & Law, 2002).

The reader is instead encouraged to ask: How should we understand this complexity? What are the constituents? Accordingly, the chapters do not fit into one complete and coherent story. Some of the chapters present reactions or even solutions to problems enhanced by COVID-19. However, we do not offer a common grand solution based on these suggestions. This is not a weakness; it is a strength. At the beginning of the pandemic, Mol and Hardon (2020) advised scholars to look beyond the conception of interdisciplinarity as a way of combining pieces of a jigsaw puzzle. They write: '[... ...] interdisciplinarity, if it is to prove worthwhile, is not a matter of addition, but of negotiation. It thrives on attention to the concerns raised by each and every relevant discipline' (Mol & Hardon, 2020). Following this, we value the fact that each chapter can be read as an invitation to find solutions together, in ways where each analysis still follows its own path or trajectory. This invitation is continuous and also reaches out to the readers. One could say that the chapters coexist. The project of the book is infinite. More chapters could be added, as long as they are also understood as invitations to further reflection.

The structure of the edited collection

Through a collection of chapters, divided into four parts, the book presents interdisciplinary perspectives on: (i) societal reactions to the crisis, (ii) the impact on everyday life when the crisis hit, (iii) how urgent changes were introduced and how these may contribute to sustainable developments in the welfare state, and (iv) how history and the development of knowledge can provide us with insights for a better understanding of future crises and transformations.

Societal reactions: Communication and legitimacy in a time of crisis

The COVID-19 crisis is the contemporary epitome of a crisis that changed the social fabric of societies. The health crisis entailed important changes in people's everyday lives. This crisis is neither the first nor the last in contemporary society, and it presents aspects from which societies can learn. Communication from politicians and scientists was strengthened with the argument that informing and guiding the public was crucial. Restrictions formerly perceived as unthinkable were introduced and legitimised in various ways. Different formats of risk communication and crisis communication were at play; most, but not all, countries decided on recommendations or laws on the use of face masks. Chapter 2, with theoretical inspiration from the ANT tradition, presents an analysis of how the face mask became a controversial actant in the communication and handling of COVID-19 in Denmark. This analysis provides insights into decisions taken in handling and communicating a pandemic crisis.

Restrictions and ultimately lockdowns became a reality in most countries in one way or another. Denmark was one of the first countries in Europe to adopt what had previously been considered an extreme measure. Inspired by a theoretical approach to biopolitics, Chapter 3 suggests an analysis of how the new measures were legitimised by the authorities. The analysis emphasises the importance given to the moral dimension of the arguments presented, which stresses the ideal of shared 'social-mindedness' as a grand solution to the many risks caused by COVID-19. Chapter 4 explores how the biopolitical state searched to protect its citizens from a normative ethical perspective. It presents an analysis of how basic ethical principles of autonomy, dignity, integrity, and vulnerability in protecting the human person become important in bioethics and biolaw in times of the Anthropocene.

People and everyday life: Intimacy and care when the crisis hits

People were faced with strict restrictions in their everyday lives due to the crisis. They became isolated during the lockdown and had to invent new ways of engaging in social life. Chapter 5 highlights how the crisis also created new opportunities and ways of participation and inclusion for children who were already socially isolated due to their impairments. The chapter proposes insights into how the lived citizenship of disabled children and young people can be improved due to the new COVID-19 experiences of the children and youth interviewed. Chapter 6 illustrates how the crisis strengthened already existing ageing abjection and thus reflects upon a possible nuanced understanding of vulnerability. Older people were at particular risk of experiencing increased loneliness. Finally, Chapter 7 challenges the normative expectations of cohabitation, which assume physical proximity as an essential condition of intimate relationships. The chapter investigates how LATT (living apart together transnationally) couples managed to maintain a level of intimacy in a pandemic.

Urgent changes and sustainable solutions: Crisis as a gamechanger for sustainable development?

The COVID-19 crisis caused an urgent need for organisations and institutions to adapt within a very short time frame, either to prevent the spread of the virus or to fulfil their role in the provision of health care. At the same time, the crisis created a window of opportunity for change to take place and thus contribute to a sustainable development of the welfare state. The chapters in this section explore this topic from four different perspectives. Chapter 8 explores how health professionals experienced changes in interprofessional collaboration during COVID-19. The analysis shows how new and flexible collaborations emerged, and discusses whether the traditional professional boundaries will be re-established in the post- pandemic health care system. Chapter 9 investigates the changes that needed to be urgently developed and implemented in health care, with a particular focus on digital support for clinical work practices. The chapter analyses the factors that enabled and constrained these change processes and what consequences can be derived to support urgent change during possible future crises. Chapter 10 explores the causes of multiple outbreaks of COVID-19 in the meat industry during the crisis and analyses how this may lead to the sustainable development of this industry. Chapter 11 offers a perspective of public governance. The chapter explores possible alterations of policies related to achieving the United Nations (UN) 17 sustainable development goals and how these can be addressed through new policies, governance, and planning initiatives in the wake of the COVID-19 crisis.

Development of knowledge: Scientific changes in epidemiology and microbiology and lasting effects

Development of knowledge has proven to be essential in the management of crises. Chapter 12 reviews the historical origins of the pillars of mitigation in public health (isolation, quarantine, hygiene, sanitation, and vaccination), which were essential for coping with the COVID-19 crisis. As the chapter demonstrates, the historical framework in conjunction with insights from modern epidemiology provides fundamental knowledge of how to respond to future crises. Chapter 13 describes how the importance of microbes in the gut has been acknowledged since the 17th century. Exploring the hypothesis that COVID-19 has affected the human gut microbiota in several ways, the chapter emphasises that knowledge needs to be developed on how crises such as pandemics, economic crises, and climate changes influence the gut microbes and thus health.

Although these various chapters and analyses stem from a specific Danish context, in her epilogue to this edited collection Professor Deborah Lupton emphasises two important learning potentials for the future. First, the analyses resonate with how the crisis was experienced in similar wealthy countries globally and thus highlight the vulnerability of health maintenance and health promotion. Second, the analyses also highlight the importance of setting health provision and health promotion on the political agenda of the welfare state.

References

Barry, A., Born, G., & Weszkalnys, G. (2008). Logics of interdisciplinarity. *Economy and Society*, *37*(1), 20–49.

Conrad, J. (2002). Limitations to interdisciplinarity in problem oriented social science research. *The Journal of Transdisciplinary Environmental Studies*, *1*(1). https://journal-tes.ruc.dk/wp-content/uploads/2021/05/problem-oriented-conrad-2.pdf

Jelsøe, E., Thualagant, N., Holm, J., Kjærgård, B., Andersen, H. L., From, D.-M., Land, B., & Pedersen, K. B. (2018). A future task for health promotion research: Integration of health promotion and sustainable development. *Scandinavian Journal of Public Health*, *46*(Suppl 20). 10.1177/1403494817744126

Kueffer, C., Underwood, G., Hirsch Hadorn, R., Holderegger, M., Lehning, C., Pohl, M., Schirmer, R., Schwarzenbach, M., Stauffacher, G., Wuelser, G., & Edwards, P. (2012). Enabling effective problem-oriented research for sustainable development. *Ecology and Society*, *17*(4), 8.

Mol, A., & Hardon, A. (2020). What COVID-19 may teach us about interdisciplinarity. *BMJ Global Health*, *5*(12), e004375. 10.1136/bmjgh-2020-004375

Mol, A., & Law, J. (2002). Complexities: An introduction. In J. Law & A. Mol (Eds.), *Complexities: Social studies of knowledge practices* (pp. 1–23). Duke University Press.

Organisation for Economic Co-operation and Development (OECD). (1972). *Interdisciplinarity: Problems of teaching and research in universities*. OECD Publications Center.

Richard, L., Gauvin, L., & Raine, K. (2011). Ecological models revisited: Their uses and evolution in health promotion over two decades. *Annual Review of Public Health*, *32*, 307–326. 10.1146/annurev-publhealth-031210-101141

Rittel, H. W. J., & Webber, M. M. (1973). Dilemmas in general theory of planning. *Policy Sciences*, *4*, 155–169.

Part 1

Societal reactions

Communication and legitimacy in a time of crisis

2 Face masks in the Danish COVID-19 context

A representative of the crisis and communication strategies

Pernille Almlund

Introduction

Never have face masks received so much attention in the public sphere and the public debate in Denmark as during COVID-19. Until then, most people connected face masks to the health care system and mainly during surgery; we notice them only as we go under anaesthesia, with only a moment to ponder if the anaesthesia nurse has friendly eyes.

From the beginning of the pandemic, through the different periods when face masks were mandatory, they have been a hot topic in Denmark. This was even the case before Denmark was locked down, when the Danish Health Authority realised that personal protective equipment (PPE) such as face masks could be in short supply, as could test equipment and respirators. The public debate has been about whether there is evidence that masks have any effect, and why different countries' governments have implemented their use in very different ways and at different times. Additionally, it has been discussed why the government decided that August was the right time to introduce the mandatory use of face masks in certain situations and places in Denmark and how the masks suddenly became a tool in the authorities' toolbox, should further precautions be necessary. The debate about face masks has been prominent throughout COVID-19 and face masks are therefore a relevant 'representative' (Callon, 1986) of the debate about protective measures and the authorities' public risk communication about COVID-19.

This makes face masks 'an actant' in the sense of actants in actor-network-theory (ANT), i.e. human and non-human actors that produce a reaction in other human or non-human actors (Latour, 2005). This has certainly been the case with face masks in the context of COVID-19. They caused a variety of controversies throughout the pandemic, and these controversies can be seen to represent communication through lockdowns, re-opening, and the general tightening of measures in the attempt to keep society open despite increasing infection rates. Against the background of ANT, the analysis will follow the controversies and hence trace part of the network of face masks during COVID-19.

DOI: 10.4324/9781003441915-3

With its focus on controversies, actants, and risk communication, this study places itself in a research tradition between ANT and the sociology of risk (Andersen & Almlund, 2013; Arnoldi, 2009; Callon et al., 2009; Lupton, 1999; Rose & Novas, 2005Rose Ong 2005). In doing so, the study questions any given perceptions of risk and instead opens the field by following the controversies (Callon et al., 2009; Latour, 2005) and their disclosure of how authorities' risk perception and professional approach led to a view of the population as being irrational (Almlund, 2023; Lupton, 2013; Rose & Novas, 2005).

The chapter is divided into four sections. The first section will present the use and non-use of face masks during COVID-19 in Denmark. The second section will deal with the theoretical and methodological approach, focusing on actor-network theory, including controversies and the idea of security. The third section will present and conduct an analysis of the four most prominent controversies found in the data, and the final section will offer some concluding remarks and answer the research question: How are the authorities' strategic decisions and assumptions related to COVID-19 unravelled by following controversies about face masks in its risk communication?

When face masks became a daily experience

In some countries around the world, people wear a face covering due to air pollution or risk of infection from disease. This is especially true of Asian countries and the literature mentions this as one reason why these countries more quickly (Triukose et al., 2021) than most European countries gained control over the spread of COVID-19. In Denmark, face masks have never been widely used, not even in 2009/2010 during the threat of a swine flu pandemic (Andersen & Almlund, 2013). During COVID-19, however, light blue face masks became a common sight on the streets of Denmark, and for the first time were made mandatory in public transport on 22 August 2020 (Frederiksen, press conference, 15 August 2020), about six months after the disease had spread to Denmark.

Mandatory use of face masks was introduced in Danish airports on 5 June 2020. On 9 July, masks were also recommended in special situations such as for a suspected case of COVID-19 about to be tested (Lange, 2020). In early August, face masks were recommended, especially for elderly and vulnerable people when it was difficult to maintain the necessary distance to protect them from infection (Sundhedsstyrelsen, 2020). This recommendation phase was replaced by mandatory wearing of face masks on public transport on 22 August 2020, and a stronger recommendation for elderly and vulnerable people to wear masks in all situations where social distancing was difficult (Brostrøm, press conference, 15 August 2020). From mid-September, mandatory face masks were introduced in bars and restaurants in parts of the Copenhagen region when people were not sitting down, and this restriction was extended to the whole country on 4 October (Frederiksen, press conference, 18 September 2020). On 29 October, the mandatory wearing of face masks was extended to include indoor public spaces such as shops, hospitals, cinemas, and educational institutions (Frederiksen, press conference, 23 October 2020). In December 2020, Denmark was partially locked down, but this was less intrusive and comprehensive than the first partial lock down[1] in March 2020. The introduction of the mandatory use of face masks marked the point when the masks became part of the authorities' toolbox as an additional tool the government could use to avoid strict restrictions and lockdowns of the country (Jørgensen, 2020).

The mandatory wearing of face masks was lifted in June 2021 and in September of that year, COVID-19 was no longer designated as a critical threat to society. However, only two months later, in November 2021, COVID-19 was once again considered a critical threat and face masks again became mandatory in public transport, shops, and public institutions. Mandatory use of face masks was even extended to cover more situations such as driving tests, churches, libraries, and fitness centres in mid-December (Frederiksen, press conference, 1 December 2021; Heunicke, press conference, 17 December 2021). All restrictions were lifted on 1 February 2022 and COVID-19 was no longer designated as a critical threat to society. Only a strong recommendation for care homes and hospitals to require face masks and COVID-19 passports for visitors was retained (Heunicke, press conference, 26 January 2022).

Before face masks on public transport were made mandatory, there was considerable debate about whether they helped to prevent infection. Many other countries had already introduced face masks early in the pandemic based on the expectation that they would have an effect and on previous experience. In Denmark, the authorities announced that the effect of using face masks was not fully known, and masks could therefore provide a false sense of security (Jørgensen, 2020), which might make people neglect the more important hygiene measures and the social distancing recommendation. Further, as people were not used to wearing face masks, they might use them inappropriately, which could increase the risk of infection (Sonne, 2020).

In May 2020, Danish researchers initiated a randomised controlled trial (RCT) involving 6024 participants. The objective was to find out whether face masks protect wearers from COVID-19; the result was that face masks seemed to provide a small, but not statistically significant, degree of protection (Bundgaard et al., 2020). From the beginning, this project received considerable attention in Denmark and the authorities hoped that the study would provide positive evidence of the effectiveness of face masks to enable them to be recommended. However, the publishing of the research was postponed due to the review process and the rejection of the study by several journals (Ringgaard, 2020). When it was finally published in November 2020, it received much criticism as well as some positive reviews (Ringgaard, 2020; Sonne & Ringgaard, 2020). Some of the criticism referred to the fact that the study was conducted in May when infection rates were low in Denmark and found it strange that the study investigated how far face masks could protect the wearer, since the Danish recommendations assumed that masks were more effective in protecting others from infection. In any event, the results did not give the authorities the evidence they were looking for to support their decisions.

The Danish handling of face masks was a significant representative of Danish COVID-19 handling in general and was performed slightly differently than in other countries, including welfare states (Brostrøm, press conferences on 15 August and 7 December 2020; Folketinget, 2021; Triukose et al., 2021). This was strongly symbolised by the clear focus on the lack of evidence of a positive effect of a general use of face masks and the significant shift from no recommendations of face masks to a relatively widespread mandatory mask requirement in August 2020. Denmark followed a mainly political and state-controlled strategy, but there was still collaboration with health authorities and expertise (Almlund et al., 2023; Folketinget, 2021; Johansson et al., 2023). This strategy certainly influenced, but did not directly or unambiguously cause, the way face masks were handled; the link between strategy and handling was certainly more complex. Due to this complexity, the specific handling of face masks and Denmark's political yet interactive strategy, Denmark is the case of this study where the doings (Abrahamsson et al., 2015; Mol, 2003) with and around face masks are the representative (Callon, 1986) of Danish COVID-19 handling and performance.

ANT and security

Investigating a pandemic and all the phenomena affected by it or affecting it requires an interdisciplinary approach. The development of the virus cannot be understood solely through medical studies; one must also focus on human behaviour, traditionally explored as a social science phenomenon or within the humanities. The converse also applies; communication about COVID-19 as a traditional humanistic approach also needs to focus on, e.g., virus mutation, infection rates, and the effect of wearing face masks. This makes the actor-network-theory a relevant analytical approach since ANT does not separate scientific disciplines even though the theory is normally categorised under sociology. But as Latour has stated, it is a fundamentally different kind of sociology, being as much ontology as it is sociology (Latour, 1992, 2005).

In that sense, ANT is the epitome of interdisciplinarity, or more correctly, it is beyond interdisciplinarity, as explicitly expressed by Bruno Latour when he stated: 'We have never been modern', referring to how scientific disciplines were split up a long time ago, which he regards as very problematic (Latour, 1993). This is because such a division of disciplines fails to examine and understand phenomena, both in the past and the future, as an outcome of multiple and mixed processes, not delimited by traditional scientific disciplines. Examples of multi-faceted phenomena which are having problematic consequences include climate change, loss of biodiversity, and zoonosis.

ANT analysis does not distinguish between theory and methodology. This is because ANT involves tracing a network in an attempt to follow the dynamic relations between human and non-human actants with the objective to understand a phenomenon and its co-creative influence on society at the specific time of the investigation. In the ANT approach, we will never start with a description of how society appears, with, e.g., structures or categories to explain the dynamic relations – it is done in the reverse order, with a switch between foreground and background as they have traditionally been understood (Blok & Jensen, 2009). This covers both methodology and theory, including practical and philosophical directives in science and ontology (Latour, 1992, 2005; Mol, 1999, 2003).

To initiate a network analysis means to choose a 'primum movens', which is the actant selected as the point of departure for the analysis (Callon, 1986). In this specific analysis, face masks are the primum movens, because they are crucial for the understanding of risk and crisis communication in Denmark. To trace the face mask network is then to follow this non-human actant's relations to other human and non-human actants. With an ANT approach, the objective is to find and follow all relations, since all actants are equal and we cannot understand the importance of each of them if any of them are overlooked. Obviously, this is a very ambitious goal and unfeasible within the time constraints of a traditional research project (not least because the dynamicity continues infinitely), but as an approach and a source of inspiration it can still ensure that we take a descriptive approach without resorting to predetermined explanations.

In tracing a network, both Callon and Latour focus specifically on relations which can be deemed to be controversies, because controversies leave empirical traces. In ANT, controversies can be understood and defined as anything from small disputes and discussions to regular conflicts, but they are all easy to follow due to their visible footprints (Callon et al., 2009; Latour, 2005). Therefore, to trace a network also involves identifying and following controversies and tracing a full network can even be replaced by an approach tracing only controversies, which is the approach in this study.

Controversies are expressed through communication, if communication is understood broadly as being verbal, written and body language; in this way, controversies leave empirical tracks via communication. Thus the controversies we are interested in will be identified and followed through communication expressed in all articles published by *Videnskab.dk* in 2020, 2021, and 2022[2] that discuss and/or present aspects of face masks (34 out of 138 articles mentioning face masks are included), all 26 press conferences held by the government in 2020, 2021, and the first one in 2022 as a result of COVID-19, and a letter from the Danish Medicines Agency to the distributors of medical equipment in Denmark, but not through a more traditional sample of media texts in general. This empirical sample was selected as the most direct exponent of controversies related to the authorities and the contemporaneous political and professional strategy of the use of face masks, with *Videnskab.dk* representing a large number of professional voices and discussions, the press conferences representing the most initial and direct political and professional collaboration and strategy and the letter representing one example of the health authorities' internal voice, which I came across by accident when I was asked by a journalist from the Danish newspaper Politiken to comment on the letter.

By following the relational work of face masks (Mol, 1999, 2003), the texts were then read and scrutinised for the presence of controversies and to determine whether these controversies constituted some sort of thematic pattern (Braun & Clarke, 2006; Kvale & Brinkmann, 2015; Latour, 2005). The data are then coded by identifying and tracking controversies; this replaces a more traditional qualitative categorisation of the data but is still systematic and comprehensive. When each small dispute or disagreement can be a controversy, hence each combination of a question and an answer can be a controversy, one way to achieve an overview was to be aware of and produce thematic groupings of controversial statements. In this process, the four most prominent controversies were identified, although a few others were found that were not so prominent in the data. Among these were the safety of face masks made of fabric compared to medical face masks, how to handle the 'covering prohibition law'[3] in combination with mandatory use of face masks, and environmental issues related to the use of such a huge amount of disposable masks.

The objective was to identify all controversies about face masks and then focus on those that tell us most about the general trends and the basis for the authorities' risk and crisis communication. In general, controversies express some sort of insecurity,[4] but insecurity will also be dealt with in the focus on controversies (Callon et al., 2009; Latour, 2005). In this way, an ANT approach is linked to a risk or insecurity perspective, hence we gain a risk and crisis communication perspective.

In line with the idea of not initiating an analysis with given concepts and categories and writing out the controversies, each of them is presented in a narrative way and followed by a theoretical summary. Such a narrative presentation is in accordance with ANT, in its ambition to emphasise the descriptive and tight analytical approach and appreciate the researcher as the mediator of the investigation (Latour, 2005).

Analysis

What has been remarkably absent in the public debate about face masks in Denmark is how the use of masks covering the face is incompatible with the 'covering prohibition law' (see endtnote 3) in Denmark, introduced back in 2018 as an expansion of the mask prohibition law from 2000. Only one of the articles from *Videnskab.dk*, written by two researchers from Roskilde

University, involves the question of whether this law was a reason for the late introduction of face masks in Denmark, and they postulate how it might have been important to keep the Danish name for face masks, translated literally as 'mouth pads', thereby avoiding the word 'mask' in this context[5] (Riis & Pedersen, 2021). The absence of any debate is remarkable because this law was hotly debated and led to many protests in Denmark, especially because the expansion in 2018 was perceived to be controversial, since the prohibition also includes people wearing *burkas* and *niqabs*. The law was informally called the 'burka ban'. Paragraph 3 of Section 134 b states: 'The prohibitions mentioned in paragraphs 1 and 2 do not concern face coverings which serve a practical purpose', and the absence of any debate may of course indicate that the media and debaters in general had accepted that face masks were intended to serve a practical purpose.

In contrast to this absence of public debate, other perspectives and controversies on face masks figured strongly in the debate. The analysis focuses on the four most prominent controversies which, as mentioned earlier, do not constitute an exhaustive list of all controversies about face masks. These controversies are (1) the debate surrounding the possibility of a shortage of face masks, (2) citizens' ability or inability to handle information on face masks and use them appropriately, (3) a discussion on how evidence differs from experiences of the effects of wearing face masks, and (4) face masks as a tool in the government's toolbox of measures.

The debate surrounding the possibility of a shortage of masks

Like many other nations, Denmark had a shortage of PPE, including face masks, when COVID-19 reached the country. This was known even before the government realised that it would probably also hit Denmark (Folketinget, 2021). On 27 February, *Videnskab.dk* wrote that face masks were sold out in many places and were being sold at inflated prices over the Internet. They quoted Brian Kristensen, a section leader from the State Serum Institute (SSI)[6] as saying: 'The number of face masks is not unlimited, and this is why we recommend saving the masks for the people who need them and who know how to use them'.

At a press conference on 6 March 2020, a journalist opened by commenting that people at that time were hoarding face masks and that suppliers reported that they would probably not be able to fulfil all orders for hand sanitisers. To a follow-up question regarding the lack of plastic for test kits, Brostrøm answered:

> We are in very, very close dialogue with the regions and hospitals and other parts of the health care system about these challenges. With the Danish Medicines Agency, we are looking for storage capacity in Denmark, delivery options and any possible supply problems. We are looking at our entire capacity. And this includes test kits and protective equipment for staff.

> The journalist then asked: 'But is there a problem?' Brostrøm answers: 'Globally there are some general supply challenges, including for test kits, but we are quite optimistic that we will be able to manage in Denmark' (Press conference, 6 March).

As part of this investigation into storage capacity and delivery options, on 5 March, the day before the press conference, the Danish Medicines Agency had sent out a letter to all suppliers of medical equipment in Denmark with advice on how to prioritise supplies of equipment, etc. for the Danish health care system. The most remarkable part of the letter was the end, where suppliers were encouraged to handle this enquiry with caution:

> The Danish Medicines Agency would ask you to handle this inquiry with some caution and not create unnecessary fear in the population about a possible lack of protective equipment due to the outbreak of COVID-19. Therefore, please inform us prior to sending out any communication or press releases. (Danish Medicines Agency, 5 March 2020)

This letter was later leaked to the Danish newspaper Politiken, which might have been expected by the health authorities, since a disclosure of secrets will always be relevant for the media. In this case, the health authorities' attempt to treat this as a secret could even have given citizens a reason to remain suspicious and uncertain. This leak did not cause any strong reaction, but it is an indication of the health authorities' communication during COVID-19 and how they perceive the general public.

Bearing in mind Brostrøm's optimism at the press conference of 6 March, the shortage of face masks was more explicitly mentioned and debated as problematic at the following press conferences. Both the chairman of KL – Local Government Denmark,[7] Jacob Bundsgaard, and the chairman of Danish Regions,[8] Stephanie Lose, made it clear at a press conference on 23 March how their organisations were working hard to secure sufficient PPE at that time (Press conference, 23 March). Here, the Danish health minister talked about private donations of face masks and thanked the Danish business community for their support, which in some cases involved converting production to making face masks.

At the press conference of 6 April, the Prime Minister Mette Frederiksen stated that it was still difficult to ensure a supply of PPE and that it was a problem that front-line staff did not have the right equipment. *Videnskab.dk* also discussed the problematic situation on 7 April: 'At the moment there is a lack of protective equipment for health staff in Denmark, and this has been cited as the reason why face masks are not yet recommended for all Danes'. They continued by quoting Brian Kristensen of SSI, who rejected the implication that the lack of face masks was the reason for that decision: 'I am not familiar with the supply situation in general, but all our recommendations are based exclusively on sound scientific documentation'.

The debate and controversy about the lack of face masks and PPE, in general, came to an end at the press conference on 12 May 2020. By this time, Denmark was well supplied with face masks and PPE, and the press conference was primarily held to inform the nation about plans to strengthen emergency measures by establishing a new committee to ensure supplies and stocks of PPE, test kits, and isolation facilities for future emergencies. The prime minister stated how important it was to prioritise sufficient supplies of equipment: 'The next step is to build up stocks for the coming summer and autumn and for the future. We need to be ambitious. We now consider protective equipment as critical infrastructure for society'. These final words suggest that Denmark, like most other nations, was ill prepared for a pandemic like COVID-19 and that the government wanted Danish society to be well prepared for future pandemics. This controversy has thus clearly had a learning outcome, which will probably be of benefit in the next pandemic situation.

We see here how face masks as a 'representative actant' (Latour, 2005) show us an important aspect of the Danish handling of COVID-19 or more specifically the handling of the risk of being in short supply of important equipment. The debate on this handling did not become problematic due to the risk of insufficient equipment and the authorities' unpreparedness, but due to the authorities' attempt to hide this shortage. This intention to hide the shortage suggested a perception of Danes as being governed by their emotions, unable to think rationally in such a crisis. This perception of the general public has also been observed in other high-stakes situations (Almlund, 2023; Lupton, 2013).

Citizens' inability

As already mentioned, two reasons that face masks were neither recommended nor required in general was that they could provide a false sense of security and that people would probably be unable to use them appropriately. *Videnskab.dk* had already quoted Brian Kristensen of the SSI on 27 February 2020 as saying: 'Masks or mouth pads can even have the opposite effect or directly spread infection if they are not used correctly', and he continued: 'If a mask or a mouth pad is contaminated with the virus, the outside of the mask can be a source of infection if people do not take them off and discard them properly'.

In another article in *Videnskab.dk* on 7 April 2020, after interviews with Clinical Professor Henning Bundsgaard and Brian Kristensen of the SSI, a journalist summed up as follows:

> We do not know how the Danes will use face masks, and therefore it is not clear if the face masks will have the desired effect. In the worst case, the face masks will lead to a false sense of security, so the argument goes.

At the press conference on 15 August 2020 when mandatory wearing of face masks in public transport was presented, a journalist referred to these arguments, asking whether face masks had any effect if people did not use them correctly. In his rather long question, he referred to a video where the director of the National Board of Health, Søren Brostrøm, demonstrates the correct use of face masks in a sterile room and encouraged Brostrøm to demonstrate the use in a non-sterile room such as the one they were in.

Søren Brostrøm took up the advice and said after the demonstration: 'It obviously looks elegant when I do this, because I have 20 years' experience.[9] I realise that other people do not have that. I just think that we should all work on that, Brian (the journalist, ed.). I also noticed you did not cough in accordance with the guidelines from the National Board of Health. I can show you that afterwards.' He continued:

> That is a really good question. There is no doubt that if people do not wear the face mask correctly, it will not have the same effect or the high effect. If people wear it completely wrongly, it may do more harm than good. From an overall perspective, if we all use face masks, and most people do it more or less correctly, then we will have a preventative effect. And that is what has been seen in other countries' experience.

Regarding the risk of people having a 'false sense of security', which could make them more lax about other restrictions, Søren Brostrøm made a reference to studies showing that wearing face masks seemed to remind people about other restrictions at the press conference on 15 August 2020. This new knowledge was underlined by *Videnskab.dk* on 2 November 2020, referring to a study showing that people still try to comply with other restrictions when wearing face masks. This observational study showed that it was crowding that dictated compliance with restrictions, not lax behaviour.

Again, we find face masks as a comprehensive representative actant (Callon, 1986), here showing the authorities bipolar perception of face masks, when inner contamination and outer contamination express face masks as two different materialities (Mol, 2003). Used by health care personal, the contamination is kept correctly on the inside, while in the hands of incapable citizens, it is expected to be wrongly on the outside. This invisible shift from right to wrong contamination makes 'a false sense of security' and 'the lack of preventative effect' important actants in this controversy. This bipolar perception changed from first tipping towards the fear of outside contamination to tipping towards trust in people's ability to keep the contamination on the inner side.

Evidence or experience

As already mentioned, a search for evidence has been prominent in discussions on the strategy for handling the COVID-19 crisis in general and face masks in particular. As early as 27 February 2020, *Videnskab.dk* referred to a systematic review that found that face masks were effective when used by health staff and infected people and may also have a small effect in the general population if combined with other hygiene measures, but the overall conclusion was that this field was greatly understudied.

At the press conference on 6 March 2020, one journalist asked if people should not just start wearing masks. Søren Brostrøm replied: 'Regarding face masks, there is no evidence that they prevent infection. So what you see in Asian countries, that is a strong cultural tradition – we do not recommend everyone to wear face masks'.

Videnskab.dk highlighted on 7 April 2020 that the health authorities still did not recommend face masks despite their use in other countries. They also mentioned that laboratory experiments showed how a face mask could reduce the virus in the air around the person wearing it. Brian Kristensen of the SSI was quoted as saying: 'We do not disagree that face masks work in a laboratory. We know that. But we have no evidence that they work in public spaces, so we do not recommend them'. This was also underlined by Henning Bundgaard and it was mentioned that he would initiate an RCT among Danes in May. This is the study already described in the background section.

A similar question was posed at the press conference on 12 May 2020 and a similar reply was given by Brostrøm: 'But a general recommendation that we should all wear face masks when we leave the house is not part of our toolbox at present'.

Another journalist asked at the same press conference if the authorities throughout the past three months had designed the guidelines based on the amounts of PPE available. Søren Brostrøm replied:

> We do of course take many considerations into account when we design our professional guidelines. Primarily, what is the evidence in the field. What practical experience is there, what is practically possible, and of course our guidelines have to consider the real-life situation. So, we have made guidelines about rational use of protective equipment. We had to do that because we could see we had a shortage. So, we have to give the health care system and the staff some guidelines for their priorities.

On 31 July 2020, *Videnskab.dk* published an article quoting Chief Physician Jens Lundgren, who pointed out various reasons to recommend face masks. New real-life studies had shown that face masks have an effect and new knowledge about the behaviour of the virus could support the use of face masks. The new knowledge at that time was that the virus did infect others even if the infected person was asymptomatic, and that infection depended on the amount of virus particles inhaled. Lundgren was quoted as saying: 'You will not get infected if you only inhale one virus particle, but it is the concentration of virus that is important, and face masks can help to minimise this'.

Some of this knowledge may have encouraged the government to change its recommendations and begin to recommend face masks in specific situations and at the press conference on 15 August 2020 introduce mandatory face masks in public transport from 22 August. Now the authorities faced journalists who questioned the effect and evidence of face masks. At this press conference Brostrøm replied: 'Unfortunately, we do not have perfect scientific evidence. We would like to have big randomized experiments, well, we haven't got any, but we have enough documentation to consider it'.

The journalists also referred to the health authorities' earlier point that people may be unable to use masks correctly and that they may provide a false sense of security. Brostrøm's reply was: 'We have got more knowledge, although it is not perfect. We have gained some experience from abroad and we must act on it'. Later in the press conference, he said:

> I think you must realise that documentation is never black and white. And what we follow here for single-use face masks, which is well documented, but also for fabric face masks, which are less well documented, maybe do not have the same degree of filtration, is that all else being equal, a mask is better than no mask.

On 14 September 2020, *Videnskab.dk* mentioned more new studies to underline the effect of using face masks. Face masks seemed to reduce infection and laboratory experiments indicated a reduction of up to 90% of virus particles. However, the need for more large real-life RCTs was also underlined.

At press conferences on 18 September and 7 December, journalists raised questions about the effect of face masks, mentioning how Brostrøm did not recommend masks in the spring and why mandatory face masks was not expanded as in other countries. Brostrøm commented on these questions at both press conferences. On 7 December, he replied:

> We know things from foreign countries, and face masks is a very good example where we changed our position, because we were convinced by documentation. It was foreign data; we did not have any experience with face masks. But there was for instance Germany, which had introduced face masks in some places before others.

Videnskab.dk also wrote about studies of the effect of face masks from 2020 to 2022 and mentioned criticism that not more RCTs have been funded and prioritised. Examples of articles in 2021 are on 22 March, 28 May, 9 September, and 30 December 2021 and 21 February 2022. RCTs are generally in demand because of their high position in the so-called pyramid of evidence (Bhatti et al., 2006; Hansen & Henningsen, 2019; Krejsler, 2013).

It is worth noting here how evidence was originally a requirement by the government, yet they were later satisfied with imperfect documentation and experience. Experience was thus emphasised as important for the introduction of face masks since there had apparently been insufficient RCTs.

Face masks are here seen as an obvious representative of making us aware of how evidence and experience were a key controversy in the handling of COVID-19. We could even see how this led to a conflict between the government and the health authorities (Folketinget, 2021), such as at the press conference on 15 March 2020, when several journalists referred to Brostrøm's statement in the press that the lockdown and border closure were not based on a professional assessment, and then asked Prime Minister Mette Frederiksen if the lockdown was too harsh. Frederiksen replied:

> I'd prefer to say that what we can see other nations haven't done, we will try to do it in time. And the message from Italy to the rest of the world is: Do whatever you can!... ... And I want to repeat that if we wait for complete evidence to handle COVID-19, well then I'm convinced we'll be too late.

Face masks are thus an example of how far the health authorities would take the argument about evidence and how this ultimately could be disturbed by other countries' experience and maybe by the government's strategy. The important learning outcome is to see how evidence is unambiguously the primary factor, even in its absence, compared to the strong presence of experience. From August, experience became an argument, but only on the excuse of the lack of evidence (Bhatti et al., 2006; Krejsler, 2013).

An expansion of the toolbox

Recommendations on using face masks and mandatory face masks in airports had already been introduced in May and June, but these were not mentioned as a tool in the toolbox until late July. In *Videnskab.dk* on 31 July, a journalist called face masks a tool in the toolbox when summing up a point from Professor Jens Lundgren: 'Jens Lundgren also stresses that face masks will always only be one of several tools in the toolbox'. Later in the article the journalist also mentioned the origin of the toolbox metaphor:

> Despite powerful evidence that face masks can be effective in preventing infection, that does not mean that they will be used in Denmark – yet. The government does not recommend face masks in the public in general, even though they were announced as part of the toolbox.

Further, Thomas Benfield, a professor at Hvidovre Hospital was quoted in the article and an interview with Søren Brostrøm in Danish Radio was mentioned to describe how they both claimed that it was too early to introduce a wider use of masks, but if the infection rate increased, and it became difficult to maintain distance, it could be relevant. Moreover, Michael Bang Petersen, a professor at Århus University was quoted as saying:

> From a political perspective, I presume that the authorities will go far to avoid a lockdown again. That means they will use all possible means to avoid that. So it will be difficult not to use face masks to a greater or lesser degree.

This dual strategy of using face masks to prevent infection and to avoid a strict lockdown is what is meant by referring to a tool in the toolbox.

At the press conference on 15 August, when the mask requirement in public transport was introduced, we see how this expansion of the toolbox was part of the strategy. At this meeting, arguments for introducing face masks were presented by both Mette Frederiksen and Søren Brostrøm. Against this background, a journalist asked: ' ... why on earth didn't we start using them a long time ago?' The prime minister gave a long answer, the essence of which was: 'It's connected to the answer I gave before – that is that we make the efforts we consider to be right at the right time'.

The discussion continued and another journalist asked if any kind of standards had been set for the infection rate or other things that had now led to mandatory face masks, and when it would then be the right time to stop again. Brostrøm answered: 'There are no clear boundaries. It wouldn't make sense either. We'll always have a holistic view. But there we will include many elements'. He mentioned here how much contact is seen, movement in public places, public transport, shops, infection rate, number of newly infected, and continued by saying:

> And as already mentioned by the prime minister, you can well imagine expanding the requirement to other parts of social life. And it is also part of our toolbox to imagine that we might use face masks in more situations in local outbreaks and local situations.

Later in the press conference, Mette Frederiksen underlined: 'But I must say too, that politically our promise to Danish employees and Danish companies is that we will go far to avoid a lockdown like the one we saw in March'.

As mentioned, an expansion of the requirement to wear face masks was introduced in stages in autumn 2020 and the dual strategy continued. At the press conference on 23 October 2020, Brostrøm stated: 'So we must look at the restrictions we introduced in mid-September. Therefore, it makes good professional sense to expand them, but it also makes good health sense to tighten some of them. We have some buttons now, and we know what works'. He continued by emphasising the dual strategy as follows: 'And it's our job as health authorities to advise on actions which on the one hand we know will help us control the pandemic … but on the other hand will enable us to keep society open'.

More than a year later, at a press conference on 8 December 2021 a journalist asked Mette Frederiksen how she can continuously argue that we are in a better situation than in December 2020 now when infection rate is high, and the health care system is under pressure. She replied: 'It is still true that the vast, vast majority of society's activities are open. There are some restrictions, you could say, related to the COVID-19 passport and the use of face masks, but society is fundamentally open, and that is due to the vaccines'.

From the moment that face masks became a tool in the toolbox they also became a button that could be turned up and down, hence a clear indicator of the severity of the threat from the virus at that specific moment. None of the other tools, such as tests and vaccines, could take the place in the toolbox as such a sensitive indicator. Therefore, face masks, as the most sensitive tool, became the right tool to introduce in August 2020 based on experience, not evidence. This is one more reason why face masks became a strong and informative representative (Callon, 1986) of the authorities' strategy of handling COVID-19.

Concluding remarks

This perspective on the story of face masks in the Danish crisis and risk communication regarding COVID-19 through the lens of ANT does not involve any intention to pinpoint causal explanations for how the decision-making process took place. In following the controversies, it is more relevant to point out the relationship between them and to underline the logics they are based on.

There is no doubt that the most discussed and prominent of the controversies highlighted here is that between evidence and experience, but this is still not the only reason for not introducing mandatory wearing of face masks or at least a recommendation of using face masks in general. The focus on evidence instead of experience is strongly related to the perception that people will probably use face masks inappropriately, since there is no evidence that they are able to use them correctly. However, there seemed to be evidence for, or at least experience of, the effect of face masks among health professionals, which is related to the decision to reserve the limited supply of PPE (except sanitisers) to health care workers. In that way, the shortage is also connected to the controversy between evidence and experience. Further, when the health authorities tried to withhold the information about the shortage from the public, with the purpose to avoid panic in the population, it was related to the perception or expectation that people could not use face masks appropriately. Citizens are perceived as being emotional and not readily willing to adjust (Almlund, 2023; Lupton, 2013), despite all the adjustments taking place at that time. The widening of the toolbox, the last controversy highlighted here, is also built on the fact that some evidence of an effect of face masks and considerable experience from abroad, especially from comparable countries appeared during summer 2020. Denmark was also at that time in a situation where the supply of PPE was ample, hence it was a realistic time to introduce the mandatory wearing of face masks and different recommendations for face masks.

In relation to this 'widening of the toolbox', it is important to bear the actual situation in mind. The infection rate was rising and was expected to rise even more in the autumn and the authorities needed to find one or more additional tools to prevent the infection rate from rising too much but at the same time keep society open and productive and avoid a strict lockdown. At this time face masks became the most prominent additional tool just as tests did earlier, and still were important, while the vaccine would later become by far the strongest tool. Moreover, face masks were introduced as the most sensitive tool which could relatively easily be tuned up and down in relation to the infection rate. However, the purpose of the additional tool and the decision to use it could still not be based on strong evidence. This indicates how the controversy between evidence and experience is far from unambiguous (Bhatti et al., 2006; Krejsler, 2013), and how other perspectives must also have been part of the decision-making process (Folketinget, 2021).

We never saw any discussions of evidence, non-evidence, or experience regarding other restrictions. This indicates that other perspectives were also in play in the decision-making process. We already know from the battle between the government and the health authorities (Almlund et al., 2023; Folketinget, 2021) that political decisions were a significant part of the decision-making process, hence the crisis and risk communication, but other perspectives such as possible culturally based perspectives have been more hidden. For example, avoiding a curfew in Denmark, despite a strong infection rate, could well have a cultural explanation. Such other perspectives could be just as important to consider in the risk and crisis communication but were largely hidden behind the discussions of evidence – maybe even from the authorities themselves.

One such perspective could be the importance of trust and confidence. Traditionally, Danish society is perceived as a high-trust society where the citizens have great trust and confidence in authorities (Warren et al., 2021). However, this study has shown how trust and confidence in the opposite direction was more limited when the authorities did not trust people's ability to use face masks properly and expected them to be governed by their emotions. We have also seen how this mistrust to people's abilities transformed into trust in these very same abilities, which was necessary in the introduction of face masks as a tool in the toolbox.

In a similar way, trust in people's willingness to be vaccinated was important and necessary when vaccines later were introduced as a tool in the toolbox. The story of trust or mistrust in vaccines in Denmark is long, but in relation to COVID-19 vaccines the authorities have been more informative about possible side effects than with previous vaccines such as the HPV vaccine and the Pandemrix vaccine given in the swine flu pandemic (Senderovitz, 2021). This time the authorities based their information on their earlier experience of mistrust among citizens and this strategy seemed to be highly effective in trust building.

What we, or more correctly the authorities, can learn from this study is that they could advantageously operate on a basis of higher trust and confidence in people's abilities and benevolence in general, handle any mistrust through dialogue and in that way raise their general confidence in people's abilities, and hence raise mutual confidence.

Notes

1 In all press conferences, the first relatively comprehensive lockdown of Denmark was referred to as a partial lockdown, compared to lockdowns in other countries. One measure mentioned to underline the difference was that many other countries had introduced a curfew.
2 Videnskab.dk presents itself as Denmark's leading scientific medium. Videnskab.dk has a publishing profile and is written and edited by an independent editorial staff. Its goal is to engage with people in society, especially young people. https://videnskab.dk/om
3 This criminal law, § 134 b states that any sort of face covering preventing a person being identified in the public sphere can result in a fine or imprisonment.
4 Insecurity is the concept preferred by Callon et al. because they found the concept of risk to be strongly connected to a traditional and causal understanding.
5 The word 'mask' was not used in campaigns and official written communication, maybe because Danes traditionally use the word 'mouth pad', but it was often used by politicians and officials at press conferences.
6 About SSI: the State Serum Institute (SSI) is under the Danish Ministry of Health. Its main duty is to ensure preparedness against infectious diseases and biological threats, as well as the control of congenital disorders. https://en.ssi.dk/about-us
7 KL - Local Government Denmark is the association and interest organisation of the 98 Danish municipalities. https://www.kl.dk/english/
8 Danish Regions is the interest organisation of the five administrative regions in Denmark. Danish Regions' overall mission is to safeguard the interests of the regions nationally and internationally. Some of the most important tasks of the organization are to safeguard regional government interests in health care, hospitals, special education, regional development, the environment and finances. https://www.regioner.dk/services/in-english
9 Søren Brostrøm was a hospital doctor before becoming the Director of the National Board of Health.

References

Abrahamsson, S., Bertoni, F., Mol, A., & Martín, R. I. (2015). Living with omega-3: New materialism and enduring concerns. *Environment and Planning D: Society and Space*, *33*, 4–19. 10.1068/d14086p

Almlund, P. (2023). Mediedebatten om HPV-vaccinen – Når bivirkninger, evidens og følelser skaber kontroverser [The media debate about the HPV vaccine: When side effects, evidence and emotions create controversy]. In P. Almlund & S. V. Knudsen (Eds.), *Offentlig kommunikation – Til, om og med borgere* [Public communication: To, about and with citizens]. Samfundslitteratur.

Almlund, P., Kjeldsen, J. E., & Mølster, R. (2023). Expressions of governance, risk and responsibility. Public campaigns in the crisis and risk management of Covid-19 in Denmark, Sweden and Norway. In B. Johansson, Ø. Ihlen, J. Lindholm, & M. Blach-Ørsten (Eds.), *Communicating a pandemic: Crisis management and Covid-19 in the Nordic countries* (pp. 121–148). University of Gothenburg. 10.48335/9789188855688-6

Andersen, N. B., & Almlund, P. (2013). Fra usikkerhed om sygdom til usikkerhed om bivirkninger. En aktør-netværksteoretisk analyse af usikkerheder om influenza A(H1N1) [From uncertainty about an illness to uncertainty about the side effects. An actor-network theory-based analysis of uncertainties about influenza A(H1N1)]. *Dansk Sociologi*, *24*(2), 35–56.

Arnoldi, J. (2009). *Risk*. Polity Press.

Bhatti, Y., Hansen, H. F., & Rieper, O. (2006). *Evidensbevægelsens udvikling, organisering og arbejdsform: En kortlægningsrapport* [A report on the development, organisation and working methods of the evidence movement]. AKF-Forlaget.

Blok, A., & Jensen, T. E. (2009). *Bruno Latour – Hybride tanker i en hybrid verden* [Bruno Latour: Hybrid thoughts in a hybrid world]. Gyldendal.

Braun, V., & Clarke, V. (2006). Using thematic analysis in psychology. *Qualitative Research in Psychology*, *3*(2), 77–101. 10.1191/1478088706qp063oa

Bundgaard, H., Bundgaard, J. S., Raaschou-Pedersen, D. E. T., von Buchwald, C., Todsen, T., Norsk, J. B., Pries-Heje, M. M., Vissing, C. R., Nielsen, P. B., Winsløw, U. C., Fogh, K., Hasselbalch, R., Kristensen, J. H., Ringgaard, A., Andersen, M. P., Goecke, N. B., Trebbien, R., Skovgaard, K. Benfield, T., … Iversen, K. (2020). Effectiveness of adding a mask recommendation to other public health measures to prevent SARS-CoV-2 infection in Danish mask wearers. *Annals of Internal Medicine*, *174*(3), 335–343. 10.7326/M20-6817

Callon, M. (1986). Some elements of a sociology of translation: Domestication of the scallops and the fishermen of St. Brieuc Bay. In J. Law (Ed.), *Power, action, and belief: A new sociology of knowledge*. Routledge & Kegan Paul.

Callon, M., Lascoumes, P., & Barthe, Y. (2009). *Acting in an uncertain world: An essay on technical democracy*. The MIT Press.

Folketinget. (2021). *Håndteringen af covid-19 i foråret 2020 – Rapport afgivet af den af Folketingets Udvalg for Forretningsordenen nedsatte udredningsgruppe vedr. håndteringen af covid-19* [The handling of COVID-19 in spring 2020: A report submitted by the committee of inquiry established by the Danish Parliamentary Business Committee on the handling of COVID-19].

Hansen, H. R., & Henningsen, I. (2019). Kampen om evidens i et kritisk perspektiv [The battle for evidence in a critical perspective]. In D. D. Christoffersen & K. S. Petersen (Eds.), *Er der evidens for evidens?* [Is there evidence of evidence?]. Samfundslitteratur.

Johansson, B., Ihlen, Ø., Lindholm, J., & Blach-Ørsten, M. (2023). Introduction: Communicating a pandemic in the Nordic countries. In B. Johansson, Ø. Ihlen, J. Lindholm, & M. Blach-Ørsten (Eds.), *Communicating a pandemic: Crisis*

management and Covid-19 in the Nordic countries (pp. 11–30). University of Gothenburg. 10.48335/9789188855688-6
Jørgensen, L. B. (2020). *Brostrøm: Vi har ansigtsmasker i vores værktøjskasse.* [Brostrøm: 'We have face masks in our toolbox]. TV2.dk, 28 July.
Krejsler, J. B. (2013). 'What works' in education and social welfare? A mapping of the evidence discourse and reflections upon consequences for professionals. *Scandinavian Journal of Educational Research*, *57*(1), 16–32.
Kvale, S., & Brinkmann, S. (2015). *Interview – det kvalitative forskningsinterview som håndværk* [InterViews: Learning the craft of qualitative research interviewing]. Hans Reitzels Forlag.
Lange, F. (2020). *Nu anbefales mundbind i offentlig transport på særlige tidspunkter.* [Face masks now recommended in public transport at certain times of day]. TV2.dk, 31 July.
Latour, B. (1992). Where are the missing masses? The sociology of a few mundane artifacts. In W. E. Bijker & J. Law (Eds.), *Shaping technology/building society. Studies in sociotechnical change*. The MIT Press.
Latour, B. (1993). *We have never been modern.* Harvard University Press.
Latour, B. (2005). *En ny sociologi for et nyt samfund. Introduktion til Aktør-Netværk-Teori.* [A new sociology for a new society. An introduction to actor-network theory]. Akademisk Forlag.
Lupton, D. (1999). *Risk.* Routledge.
Lupton, D. (2013). Risk and emotion: Towards an alternative theoretical perspective. *Health, Risk & Society*, *15*(8), 634–647. 10.1080/13698575.2013.848847
Mol, A. (1999). Ontological politics. A word and some questions. *The Sociological Review*, *47*(1), 75–89.
Mol, A. (2003). *The body multiple: Ontology in medical practice.* Duke University Press.
Riis, S., & Pedersen, E. O. (2021). *Maskens vej fra forbud til påbud* [The path of face masks from prohibition to mandate]. *Videnskab.dk*, 13 May.
Ringgaard, A. (2020). *Dansk forsøg med mundbind er endt i stormvejr* [Danish face mask trial in stormy seas]. *Videnskab.dk*, 22 October.
Rose, N., & Novas, C. (2005). Biological citizenship. In A. Ong & S. Collier (Eds.), *Global assemblages: Technology, politics and ethics as anthropological problems* (pp. 439–463). Blackwell.
Senderovitz, T. (2021). *Kapløbet om vaccinen* [The race for a vaccine]. Strandberg Publishing.
Sonne, F. G. H. (2020). *Mundbind og ansigtsmasker anbefales stadig ikke til almindelige danskere* [Face masks still not recommended for ordinary Danes]. *Videnskab.dk*, 27 February.
Sonne, F. G. H., & Ringgaard, A. (2020). *"Dybt usædvanligt": Amerikanske forskere advarer mod svagheder i dansk mundbindsstudie* ['Highly unusual': American researchers warn of weaknesses in Danish face mask study]. *Videnskab.dk*, 23 October.
Sundhedsstyrelsen (2020). *Et mundbind i tasken er en god idé, når der er trængsel i den kollektive trafik* [A mask in your bag is a good idea in crowded public transport]. 31 July. https://www.sst.dk/da/nyheder/2020/et-mundbind-i-tasken-er-en-god-ide_-naar-der-er-traengsel-i-den-kollektive-trafik
Triukose, S., Nitinawarat, S., Satian, P., Somboonsavatdee, A., Chotikarn, P., Thammasanya, T., Wamlapakorn, N., Sudhinaraset, N., Boonyamalik, P., Kakhong,

B., & Poovorawan, Y. (2021). Effects of public health interventions on the epidemiological spread during the first wave of the COVID-19 outbreak in Thailand. *PLoS One*, *16*(2), e0246274.

Warren, G. W., Lofstedt, R., & Wardman, J. K. (2021). Covid-19: The winter lockdown strategy in five European nations. *Journal of Risk Research*, *24*(3-4), 267–293. 10.10 80/13669877.2021.1891802

3 Pastoral manifestations of legitimacy in a welfare state in crisis

Pelle Korsbæk Sørensen and Nicole Thualagant

Introduction

Denmark was among the first states in Europe to announce a country-wide lockdown of society in March 2020 and one of the first states to 'reopen' society in April and May 2020 (Prime Minister's Office, 2020b). Further, at the very beginning of autumn 2021, Denmark was one of the first countries in Europe to announce that the disease would no longer be categorised as a 'socially critical disease' (Danish Ministry of Health, 2021). The main argument behind this governmental decision was presented in terms of the high percentage of vaccinated citizens. This chapter is concerned with the development and legitimation of the immediate national COVID-19 response in Denmark. The scope of the analysis is theoretically inspired by biopolitics and explores how we can understand the immediate policy reaction to COVID-19 with regard to the state, social security and 'care of the self', themes questioned by Michel Foucault in his lectures on the birth of biopolitics and further developed by many Foucauldian scholars (Zamora & Behrent, 2016). We argue that the way the political responses to the crisis were legitimated is of interest in understanding how biopolitics in times of crisis is developed in a modern welfare state where health provision is essential to the legitimacy of the state.

Denmark, like other welfare states, was in a situation where not only did rapid solutions have to be provided but also solutions that needed political legitimacy. The COVID-19 situation was a new and unknown crisis that called for immediate reaction. The crisis can be understood as an exogenous shock both to society and to the individual's lifeworld. For most people, this was completely unexpected. In a welfare state in the year 2020, health was understood as a common good, as a collective and individual responsibility, and thus a shared obligation or even a moral imperative, as expressed by Deborah Lupton (1995). Michel Foucault explored in his writings how the politics of health had developed since the 18th century (Lupton, 2022, p. 61; Lynch, 2014), by highlighting how health not only became a political objective for the state in the general provision of welfare but also a state of well-being to be managed. Health became deeply interrelated with welfare. From a Foucauldian perspective, discourses are believed to reveal ideals of health, welfare, and more

DOI: 10.4324/9781003441915-4

precisely ideals of responsibilities towards the provision of health and welfare, or *welfarism* as Rose and Miller put it (Rose & Miller, 1992). Accordingly, we analyse the discourses legitimating the immediate national response to COVID-19. The scope of this chapter is to present findings relevant to the case under investigation, i.e. Denmark, yet there is a learning potential which reaches beyond the national border. In Europe and worldwide, individual states handled the crisis differently, yet there seem to be commonalities depending on the type of state and political orientation (Lynggaard et al., 2023). Denmark is particularly interesting as a welfare state with a large public workforce and a large public sector. Following Esping-Andersen's (1990a, b) typology of welfare regimes, we explore how extraordinary, rapidly implemented political measures are presented and legitimated in what Esping-Andersen describes as a universalistic social democratic welfare state. In this analysis, Denmark serves as an example of such a state.

The context of COVID-19 from a social science perspective

Since the turn of the century, we have experienced a series of crises, each with its own characteristics. The COVID-19 crisis was first and foremost a health crisis, but it soon became clear that an interdisciplinary perspective was needed. Like many other social scientists (ESA, 2021; Jensen et al., 2020; Lupton, 2022; Lynggaard, 2023), we developed a theoretical interest in understanding the different national responses to COVID-19. Different studies have informed our research question.

From a political science perspective, research describes how the government's responses to COVID-19 involved a mix of tools from several policy areas: social, health, medical, and economic. Research also highlights that the most common tools applied were economic in nature and that a strong emphasis was placed on social policy to initiate 'public health' measures (Capano et al., 2020).

Different comparative and national analyses are presented from a sociological perspective and through the theoretical lenses of governmentality or biopolitics, with a specific interest in the Foucauldian power/knowledge relationship (Constantinou, 2022).

Through a problematization approach inspired by Foucault (2007) and Bacchi (2012), scholars (Sjölander-Lindqvist et al., 2020) point out how the collective was represented as both the problem and the solution to COVID-19 in the national discourses in Germany, Italy, Spain, and Sweden. These authors refer specifically to a responsibilisation discourse in which the individual becomes the central actor. The same analysis is provided in a governmentality inspired analysis of the Swedish strategy towards COVID-19. The authors argue here that the governing of conduct and the political focus on self-management in the Swedish strategy can be understood as both a consequence of a world risk society and an enhanced ethos-politics (Nygren & Olofsson, 2020). The Swedish strategy's emphasis on and reference to epidemiology is explored as being embedded in post-materialist and postmodern values generally characterised as in opposition to modern authority, rationality, and science (Lindström, 2020). The Norwegian response to COVID-19 was analysed as an initial liberalistic response attempting to protect the market, which later in the pandemic moved towards biopolitics, where the focus was placed on public health instead (Gjerde, 2021a, 2021b). Two French researchers demonstrate how the French response to COVID-19 can be understood as an expression of biopolitical power (Maci & Duboz, 2020). In the Danish context, the concepts of power and powerlessness in relation to biopolitics have been analysed (Tønder, 2021). In addition, a historical genealogy on how epidemics were controlled in Denmark has been described via a Foucauldian approach (Fogh Jensen, 2021). Following a Foucauldian analytical path, the specific interest of this chapter is the Danish immediate policy response to COVID-19 and how the policy response was discursively legitimated with a theoretical focus on a power/knowledge relationship. The analysis is driven by a theoretical interest in how and with reference to which forms of knowledge the policy response was legitimated. We believe that this analysis is of interest since the legitimacy of the national response to the crisis potentially led to yet another problematization, namely, the approval of the state as an actor, provider, and regulator of welfare for the common good.

Why use the theoretical lens of biopolitics?

The Foucauldian concept of biopolitics seems almost inevitable in relation to the COVID-19 crisis. The concept of biopolitics invites us to conceive the population as a 'social body'. With this perspective on the population, specific attention is paid to the administration of the social body and thus how the health of the population can be governed through statistics, regulations, or vital politics. Previous analyses by the sociologist Nikolas Rose (2001a, 2001b) have emphasised how biopolitics developed through the 21st century. With a focus on how life is governed, Rose observes that health is no longer a question of the 'fitness' of the population, but is considered within two specific rationales: an economic and a moral rationale. Here Rose emphasises how biopolitics in the 21st century can be regarded as ethos-politics: individuals are made responsible for their health and are urged to develop self-techniques in the quest for performative health. The individual is no longer believed to be disciplined through a pastoral power but primarily governed by sentiments, moral nature, and guiding beliefs. Rose's observations of biopolitics in the 21st century have informed our analysis, but we also argue that our findings contribute to the theoretical approach of ethos-politics in times of crisis by illustrating how the historical pastoral form of power re-emerges as an answer to the 'problem' of COVID-19 in the discursive responses of the representatives of the Danish welfare state.

When the first lockdown came into effect at the beginning of the year 2020, most nations turned to protective measures based on national laws, citizenship, and regulation of the population living within their borders. The measures were mainly organised within the nation states. Thus, the COVID-19 situation created what could be seen as a relapse to state measures, instead of widespread international or cross-national responses to the expanding crisis. To better understand the reaction, a historical view will serve as an introduction before we start the main analysis of the way the state response was legitimised in public.

First, in a Foucauldian analysis of biopolitics, the measures and reactions can be understood in the light of the emergence of the modern state formed by biopower since the 17th and 18th centuries (Foucault, 2010). During the COVID-19 crisis, national responses were based on protecting the population in a given area. The question of the protective state runs deep in the modern history of legitimacy. The actual spread of the disease is not only a matter *for* the state, it is also a matter that problematizes the role of the state as an actor, i.e. its very legitimacy. Is it able to deliver on the contract between the people and the state? The political philosopher Thomas Hobbes described how the first steps away from the state of nature towards the modern state were based on a social contract that offered peace and security to its subjects (Hobbes, 1997). The contract offered protection from fear of harm. Some researchers and the media discussed whether the COVID-19 situation paved the way for the state to react in ways similar to the Hobbesian understanding of the uncontested sovereign (Bufacchi, 2020; Degerman et al., 2020; Oliver, 2020; Tønder, 2021). Some countries experienced a return to political measures based on a state of emergency and direct enforcement. However, based on our analysis, we argue that politics during the first lockdown in Denmark were more complex, as the sovereign state from the time of Hobbes has been replaced with an open, liberal democracy. The binary power and singular sovereignty of past centuries have been replaced with more subtle modes of governing.

Second, what we analyse is how measures were legitimated and with reference to what forms of knowledge. This calls for an understanding of the Foucauldian notion of problematization, which is closer to a rereading of current history as it unfolds than a historical analysis. In other words, it is closer to the notion of critical thinking than to the notion of genealogy to be found in Foucauldian thought (Dreyfus & Rabinow, 1982; Garland, 2014). In what proved to be very timely, Rose directly mentions how Foucault's methodological approach to illness and medicine in relation to the individual body proves its worth in relation to contemporary concerns when: '[…] disease is problematized and addressed in terms of spatial and social associations, as in the early twenty-first century concerns about Severe Acute Respiratory Syndrome (SARS) and Avian influenza' (Rose, 2007, p. 10). Those were diseases similar to COVID-19 that became pandemics. Referring to the work of Ludwik Fleck, Rose describes a methodological approach, where it is possible to analyse the emergence of a specific *style of thought*. He describes the emergence of a historically new molecular biopolitics. However, although his analysis is different from ours, we are inspired by his description of analysing a particular way of thinking, seeing and practising that includes specific *elements* where: '[...] terms, concepts, assertions, references, relations—are organized into configurations of a certain form that count as arguments and explanations' (Rose, 2007, p. 13). A specific explanation is established, and our analysis is inspired by a search for a style of thought in government statements on the crisis.

This analysis allows us to consider the present situation from a critical perspective. This leads to the research question: How was the immediate political response to COVID-19 legitimated and with references to what knowledge regimes?

The notion of political legitimacy has a long tradition in sociological and political thought (Wiesner & Harfst, 2022), such as through Weber's analyses of bureaucracy and different sources of legitimacy (Weber, 1995). We analyse the presented measures in response to the crisis and the underlying norms communicated in the actual speeches held by the authorities. Thus, we present the statements in a descriptive and analytical manner, presenting the discourses as they appear via our reading of the press conferences. We describe how the decisions are legitimised, analysing the activity of legitimation (Barker, 2001).

The empirical archive and methodology

In Denmark, at the brink of the first lockdown, a new law on the handling of epidemics was passed extremely rapidly and with full support from all parties in the Parliament. It was presented three times and passed on the same day, on 12 March 2020 (L133–2019/2020). Since it was passed unanimously, there was no reason to declare a state of emergency in Denmark. Due to the time frame, there was no time for hearings. With reference to the fast procedure, the law was passed with a so-called 'sundown clause' giving it effect for a little less than one year.[1]

As there was a very short time to prepare the law and publicly discuss its content, it is of theoretical interest to study empirically how the main actors involved in the lockdown legitimated the effects of the law and the recommendations for the public to follow. The empirical data consist of press conferences held by the Prime Minister's Office in Denmark around the time of the first lockdown. They were all televised on public television and broadcast via the website of the Prime Minister's Office. Journalists were invited to ask follow-up questions. Among those present at the press conferences were the prime minister, the minister of health, the head of police, and the head of the Danish Health Authority. Complete transcriptions are available on the website of the Prime Minister's Office, including questions and answers.

The press conferences were held most frequently just before and after the lockdown of the country, effective from 12 March 2020. Transcripts can be accessed on the website of the Prime Minister's Office (2020a). The transcriptions from each press conference are about 10 000 words in length. Our data consist of the six most important press conferences during the first wave of COVID-19. These press conferences were selected since they represent important measures introduced and explained to the public during the first wave. The first press conference selected was on 6 March 2020, while the last was on 17 March 2020. The most important briefing was held on 11 March, when the PM announced the first lockdown of Denmark due to the spread of COVID-19. Altogether, the press conferences amount to approximately 100 pages of transcripts.

The status of the empirical data is that it serves as the actual verbalisation of how the reactions to COVID-19 were legitimised by the representatives of the state, and thus the state's discursive response to the recommendations and policy in the making.

Methodological steps of the analysis

We conducted a layered analysis. The first layer was a reading of the transcripts of the press conferences similar to a thematic content analysis. We coded the material based on our first thematic analysis, and it sharpened our analysis through themes that are here presented in four complexes of legitimacy. The second reading was theoretically informed via the lens of the concept of biopolitics as framed by Foucault. This led to the key finding that the understanding of politics and morality as intertwined, as presented in the concept of biopolitics in the 21st century (Rose, 2007), was challenged. Based on this finding, we created a third layer of the analysis where one of the four complexes, the moral complex, was analysed on its own with a theoretical subset of methods based on Foucault's notion of pastoral power, as it is presented by Waring and Latif (2018). This theoretical notion led us to focus on the social techniques and technologies of the self made available to the subject as a reaction to the threat of COVID-19.

The methodological steps of the analyses are presented in Figure 3.1. The four complexes are anchored in different knowledge-power relations and are often intertwined in the statements by the actors at the press conferences.

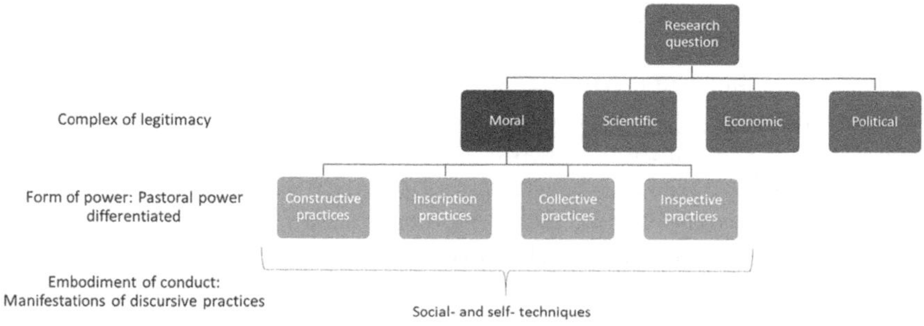

Figure 3.1 Methodological steps of the analyses.

Our findings indicate that the moral complex dominates and refer to discourses where morality as a specific form of knowledge establishes norms of conduct that are almost 'taken for granted'.

Four complexes of legitimacy

Before presenting the main findings from our analysis, this section will briefly describe the first step of the analysis, which led us to focus particularly on the moral complex through the theoretical lens of pastoral power. The analysis of the transcribed press conferences, where the initial focus was on how the political measures were legitimated, led to an exploration of arguments given for the national responses, i.e. the rationales behind the measures. The analysis of the rationales behind the national policy responses led to an identification of four main complexes of legitimacy, all overlapping when presented in the press conferences but embedded in distinct understandings of power and with reference to different knowledge regimes (Table 3.1).

One complex is *political*. The COVID-19 situation was a societal crisis, and the statements often refer to a logic based on ideas normally related to a state of emergency. However, a legal state of emergency was never declared in Denmark during the COVID-19 crisis. Instead, as described later in this chapter, the statements were based on commonality and were aimed at broad acceptance of the measures. The idea of necessity is based on arguments of being able to sustain a functioning health system under potential extreme pressure on the health system and hospitals by ill people. In political theory *the state of exception* was coined by the controversial legal and political thinker Schmitt (2007) as a situation where the sovereign decides based on the exception. In contrast, our analysis reveals that political power and implementation of measures in the modern welfare state in relation to COVID-19 needed to be explained by politicians. In a crisis, arguments can be delivered as necessary and self-explanatory in ways that might bypass an otherwise open and democratic way of presenting decisions. However, in the Danish context the measures were supported by a broad spectrum of political representation in Parliament and the measures presented during the first lockdown thus had

Table 3.1 Complex of legitimacy

Political	Arguments anchored in a political rationale as a form of knowledge that legitimates what needs to be done.
Economic	Arguments based on economics as a form of knowledge, focusing on how to balance closing down and laying off staff, especially in the public sector. Financial support packages are important here.
Scientific	Arguments based primarily on epidemiology, virology, and mathematics.
Moral	Arguments based on normative values, referring to actions to be performed individually for the sake of the common good.

broad legitimacy. Further, the legitimation of the measures was also strengthened discursively. The authorities present the measures with words such as 'necessary' and 'right', yet there is a dialogical approach in the delivery of the political messages at the press conferences where the citizens are urged to 'listen' and 'follow the recommendations' from the authorities with a strong reference to 'solidarity'. The words within quotes are from the press conference on 6 March 2020, less than one week before the first lockdown. At this press conference, the PM presents several political arguments for developing a national response to the global health crisis. It is proclaimed that a reaction from the authorities is needed and that 'everything possible' must be done to prevent the spread of the virus. The reason behind this need for an immediate response is to minimise the 'potential loss of human life' and thus, to control the as yet uncontrollable – infection by the virus. An apparatus of crisis management is installed with a strong focus on health governance. This health governance is believed to inform citizens about the virus, but also encourages certain behaviour to avoid infection. The governance of health through information on potential risks to citizens was also supported by closing the national borders and other necessary structural measures to prevent the potential spread of infection by people arriving in the country.

Another essential rationale behind the measures presented belongs to a *scientific* complex. If possible, measures and restrictions are based on scientific arguments, i.e. on a specific understanding of evidence-based knowledge. Epidemiological knowledge rapidly became the form of knowledge on which measures and restrictions were based. Epidemiology and especially knowledge about infection legitimated the restrictions and other actions, having a direct impact on people's behaviour and social life. The authorities presented new modes of behaviour to prevent the spreading of the virus and thus to have control over infection in the population. Hand hygiene, 'coughing etiquette', social distancing, and later face masks were all measures presented based on epidemiological and virological knowledge. The rationale behind the lockdown on 11 March 2020 was presented through graphs presenting two scenarios, based on a green curve and a red curve. The red curve illustrated the spread of the virus if none of the restrictions and measures were implemented or followed. The green curve illustrated the control of the spread if the measures and restrictions were followed and respected. The graph was based on mathematical models and legitimated the proposed national response. However, the curves also discursively presented two different realities. The red curve showed a health system not only under strain, but unable to keep up with demand, and thus a worst-case scenario, where the health system would be unable to provide care for all. At the press conference, this curve was often referred to as the 'Italian' situation, based on the Danes' observation of the health crisis in Italy, where the virus had severe consequences and caused many deaths among older people, possibly leading to a health system on the brink of collapse.

Another complex is *economic*. The economy was not ascribed much importance during the first days of the crisis. However, at the first press conferences, the economy is referred to in relation to two specific issues: the health system's capacity and the possible need for financial 'support packages' for specific industries and citizens. There is a stronger focus on the national economy at the press conference of 11 March where the lockdown is presented. One solution outlined is to close down some of the activities in the public sector to support the private sector. On 15 March, the economy is specifically on the political agenda, as a tripartite agreement is presented at a separate press conference. Thus, the economy, although an important complex referred to when legitimating the national response, is given less importance than the other complexes.

The moral complex appeared in our analysis to be central in the legitimation of the national response and thus overshadowed the other complexes. In the context of COVID-19, where the political focus is on the many risks caused by the virus, the risk of infection, the risk of ill health, the risk of lack of resources, and ultimately the risk of death, the strategies for managing these risks all revolve around how people behave. In fact, our analysis of the press conferences leads us to emphasise the moral dimension of the arguments behind the national response and particularly, as analysed below, an exploration of the national response as a kind of soft power installing new norms of moral conduct, in Foucauldian thought, a so-called *pastoral power*.

The Danish COVID-19 strategy as based on pastoral power relations?

The collective measures to mitigate biopolitical risks can be approached from the metaphor of pastoral power, where the focus is on the moral conduct of individuals in relation to expectations in a community (Waring & Latif, 2018). This concept is originally introduced as a metaphor by Foucault in his genealogy of governmentality, analysing Christian texts that demonstrate contemporary modes of governing the moral conduct of the 'flock'. In its historical context, pastoral power differs from traditional political power in the sense that the pastorate does not wish to govern a territory, but rather a population in constant movement. The historical objective is not to conquer land but to protect a flock. Another important difference from traditional political power to be emphasised is that the protection of the flock is given through an appeal to the individual (Foucault, 2001, pp. 551, 562). Foucault refers to four aspects that characterise pastoral power and underline the differences from traditional political power:

1 The objective of power is to lead to a common good.
2 The pastorate does not only lead, but is also willing to sacrifice itself.
3 The pastorate focuses its attention on particular individuals that constitute the 'flock'.
4 Pastoral power can only be exerted when it knows the inner world of the individual (Foucault, 2001, p. 1048).

Foucault observes a development of pastoral power in the 18th century, a new kind of institution which represents a modern state, building on elements of a pastoral power in new forms:

1 An institution where the objective of power changes. The common good becomes specified, to also involve other dimensions, such as health and well-being, protection, and security. Here medical knowledge takes on the same role that religion used to have in earlier societies.
2 The administration of pastoral power is enforced by the state or, e.g., a public institution such as the police.[2] The old idea of a central sovereign power is replaced with new institutions.
3 The new objectives and the institutions that can execute pastoral power encourage a development of specific knowledge of the individual: global, quantified knowledge of the population, and analytical knowledge of the individual (Foucault, 2001, p. 1050).

Several current researchers have drawn on the concept of pastoral power. Waring and Latif apply the concept to explore how dynamic pastoral relations are enacted in the medical encounter between patients and health professionals. They operationalise the concept by elaborating how pastoral power involves four linked practices. The first is a set of 'constructive practices', where so-called *pastors* translate governing rationalities, such as those regarding behavioural expectations, into a form that can be perceived as meaningful to the local community. A second set of practices involves 'inscription practices', where pastors discursively encourage and normalise these behavioural expectations. A third involves a set of 'collective practices', where individual behavioural expectations are related to a set of shared values of the wider community. These collective practices foster moral censure and collective reinforcement of desired behaviours. The fourth is a set of 'inspection practices', involving 'ongoing surveillance of individual and collective behaviours' (Waring & Latif, 2018, p. 1081).

The appeal to 'samfundssind' through relations of pastoral power

As developed in the above section, arguments legitimating the national response and thus the different political measures were based on different complexes: *political*, *economic*, and *scientific*. However, what our empirical analysis demonstrates is a heavy emphasis on the moral dimension of the national response and thus how restrictions and recommendations were legitimated with reference to expected moral conduct. On 10 March 2020, two days before the first lockdown, the PM introduces a concept that discursively represents this moral dimension of legitimacy. '*Samfundssind*'[3] (social-mindedness) is introduced not only as a common trait of the Danish population but also as a key solution to the crisis.

In the following we analyse how *social-mindedness* can be understood in the light of the theoretical notions of biopolitics and pastoral power. This highlights an intertwining of moral character of individual behaviour and the search for common good in the welfare society, and it displays the subtle governing of a state in a time of crisis.

The term carries values of trust and solidarity as common values in the Danish population. In the many mentions of 'samfundssind' that we identified in the empirical data, social-mindedness is often related to both individual and collective responsibility. It is emphasised that each citizen is responsible for demonstrating social-mindedness since this conduct is believed to be the key to sustainable management of the COVID-19 situation. Our analysis not only seems to support what Rose has pointed out before with the term of ethos-politics, but also permits us to contribute to the theory of ethos-politics at a time of crisis. The specific biopolitics of the 21st century in the Danish context of a global health crisis were embedded in pastoral power relations. Inspired by the work of Waring and Latif, we demonstrate through our empirical archive that a modern version of pastoral power as a technology of governance is present during a crisis.

The following analysis of the press conferences emphasises how the political response to COVID-19 can be understood as a modern form of pastoral power. As developed in the theoretical section, pastoral power involves four interrelated practices.

Constructive practices

Discourses serving as 'constructive practices' appeared in the press conferences. Several statements revealed an expectation of specific codes of conduct, such as solidarity and obedience. The PM states:

> 'Today, I would like to encourage you to practise solidarity and to encourage everyone to do what can be done regarding protection and prevention.'

Expectations of patience, courage, and care were also expressed by the PM:

> And I hope, I do understand the disappointment, I hope, that everyone, even in very specific cases, will not lose courage, and look at this from a societal perspective. There are citizens in this country who are vulnerable, and we will have to do all we can to take good care of them, and this is why, for my part, as prime minister, I appeal for social cohesion and patience.

These discourses highlighting expectations of moral conduct construct a common understanding of what is needed to manage the crisis. Through solidarity and responsibility, every citizen is believed to contribute to the management of the health crisis.

Inscription practices

Statements normalising the expected codes of conduct were also delivered, especially regarding the expectation of solidarity in relation to obedience. The PM explains:

> And with the picture we have seen until now, it is our common experience that the Danes are moving in the same direction and are taking good care of each other.
>
> But until now, I think we must say that the Danes have demonstrated a very, very, very good, very, very, very good approach to this.

The PM also emphasises how the citizens have expressed their social-mindedness:

> 'A lot of people demonstrate a fantastic sense of *samfundssind*. You must continue to do so. Because that is what works. Much of the solution to what we are facing rests on the shoulders of the Danes.'

Here social-mindedness is described as the normal conduct to follow.

Collective practices

Several statements highlight the relationship between individual behavioural expectations and the shared values of the wider community, more precisely the shared value of social-mindedness. The PM states:

> (...) but I need to emphasise that we must take more care of each other than we already have. I keep hearing some people saying: 'It won't affect me, that's why I don't care about what the authorities recommend.' You have to. Everyone has parents and grandparents. All families have people who are ill. We must take more care of them.
>
> It is a task for society – a responsibility that we all have, that we must consider seriously, that we stand together and think of other people, not only old people, but also children, all the vulnerable citizens who are extremely vulnerable to the COVID-19 virus, and therefore, once again here is a recommendation from me on behalf of the health services – show consideration, take care of each other.

These statements construct an idea of individual responsibility towards the common good and thus a reinforcement of a collective 'we', and the statements also involve a practice of moral sanctioning of those who do not demonstrate the right conduct. At some of the press conferences, the head of the police is present. The PM mentions the work of the police and social-mindedness, in the same sentences. Individual responsibility is described directly as an alternative to policing, but there is also a strong emphasis on the conduct of a small group of people not showing the politically expected form of solidarity.

> (...) the work of the police has actually been relatively easy, because there is a lot of social-mindedness out there, as such, it is a tiny minority we have to focus on (...).

> And here we are together, but there are some people who bail out of the community in the most extreme manner.

This moral argument is interesting, as it presents both a moral justification of a shared 'we' and an emphasis on individual adherence to the expected conduct.

Inspective practices

The discourses of collective practices are followed by discourses of inspective practices demonstrating ongoing surveillance. An example of this is the case of the implementation of new restrictions on crossing the national borders:

> 'But we should not take the virus from Denmark into another country. We also have a responsibility for other countries in this matter.'

Or the restriction regarding gatherings of more than a certain number of people in private homes, the PM explains:

> I would really prefer not to use the resources of the police to come round and knock on the front door of the Danes, but there are sometimes, some people who by chance hold a party with too many people and in any case with too loud music, and it is already a common task for the police to stop that.

These arguments show a subtle surveillance of conduct based on moral arguments of both individual and collective responsibility towards others' health and the shared common good.

'Samfundssind' developed through social techniques and new technologies of the self

The political statements presented above reflecting discursive practices of modern pastoral power not only shape the norms of conduct in a time of crisis, but also appeal to a self-regulated mode of conduct. This self-regulation is conducted through acts of solidarity and responsibility, but also, as will be developed further, a constant self-examination with the aim of protecting one's own health as well as the health of the social body.

As mentioned previously, Foucault explores how pastoral power takes new forms in modern institutions. More precisely, he points out that the objective of power is aimed at the common good, that the administration of pastoral power is enforced by the state and finally how pastoral power encourages the development of specific knowledge of the individual. In a pandemic context, we see the common good being secured through the political measures and the constant appeal to social-mindedness. Behaving according to a moral norm of solidarity leads to the health, protection and security of both the individual and the social body. Moreover, this aim of health, protection and security is based on quantified knowledge of the population (epidemiology, mathematics and virology) and the analytical knowledge of the individual. The constant attention to the potential risks fosters a focus on social techniques and techniques of the self (Macmillan, 2011).

Social techniques developed to prevent the risk of infection are the measures presented in terms of social relations: social distancing, coughing etiquette, hand hygiene, and later during COVID-19, face masks (see Chapter 2 on this specific measure). Social distancing is presented as an essential norm of conduct to integrate into the new normal of everyday life. This social regulation was followed by recommendations on a limited number of gatherings, home schooling and homeworking, the official suspension of handshakes, and later a recommended distance between people in social spaces.

New technologies of the self were also encouraged through the appeal to social distancing, and the general attention to hygiene. In fact, the national response encouraged a constant self-examination of potential risks and symptoms. A presentation of possible symptoms to be aware of based on expert knowledge in the press conferences urged everyone to pay attention to bodily symptoms that could potentially be a sign of infection with COVID-19. As Rose (2001a, b) presented in his earlier exploration of the politics of life itself, the development of somatic individuality encourages an approach to the body as a key site for managing the potential risks encountered in life. In the context of COVID-19, the focus on potential risks is reinforced, encouraging everyone to pay attention to potential symptoms of the virus. This increased attention to bodily symptoms emphasises the great importance attributed to the somatic individual and its compliance with moral norms of responsibility and solidarity in the pandemic welfare state. Moreover, what seems to be at stake in a time of crisis is not autonomous individuals developing techniques of the self, but rather adherent selves following the contemporary techniques of governance. The practices defining a specific mode of conduct expressed discursively in the press conferences are not just recommendations based on expert knowledge but can be understood as behavioural imperatives creating moral somatic subjects in a time of crisis.

Concluding remarks

A main finding in this study is that biopolitics at the time of the COVID-19 crisis in Denmark was developed with a predominant reference to a moral rationale, while the theory of biopolitics refers to a dominating economic rationale. However, based on the press conferences of the Prime Minister's Office, we find that the economy was not given much discursive attention when the national lockdown in Denmark in 2020 was legitimated publicly by the main actors of the state. Arguments given for the national responses to the potential health crisis were heavily based on normative expectations of moral conduct.

By analysing how the first lockdown of society was legitimated verbally by the actors present at the press conferences held by the Prime Minister's Office, we find that a moral knowledge complex was at play, and that the legitimation of the measures taken was linked to moral obligations by the individual members of society, who were to govern their actions in the light of a common aim: to make sure they would not become potential carriers of COVID-19, and thus ensure that the vulnerable members of society were not infected. In the case of Denmark, a mediating concept verbally framing this specific form of health governance is the re-emergence of the notion of *social-mindedness*. This notion is deeply rooted in a specific understanding that the right to welfare provision is linked to a specific expected conduct of the members of society, where the welfare contract is embedded in the minds of those who adhere. Finally, the appeal to samfundssind is constituted through discursive practices installing pastoral power relations between the welfare state and the social body.

Notes

1 We are fully aware that throughout this crisis there is an important dimension that refers directly to a political and administrative legitimation based on legality. Despite the importance of this, we here examine instead the statements on the implemented restrictions and strong recommendations made by the speakers at press conferences. The primary 'object' of this exploration is not the aspect of legality, rather we analyse the verbalisations and legitimations made in public via the press conferences.
2 Here the police are not to be understood directly as the police force of the present times, but as policing. There is an emphasis on the historically new regulative and pervading ways of control of the population, and the police thus represent a historical shift where power was spread out in society.
3 'Samfundssind' has been translated in the English-language press as both 'community spirit' and 'social-mindedness'. The Danish Language Council defines 'samfundssind' as 'putting the concern of society higher than one's own interests' (Gardiner, 2020). We find the term 'social-mindedness' best suited to this definition.

References

Bacchi, C. (2012). Why study problematizations? Making politics visible. *Open Journal of Political Science*, *12*(1), 1–8.

Barker, R. (2001). *Legitimating identities: The self-presentations of rulers and subjects*. Cambridge University Press.

Bufacchi, V. (2020). Coronavirus: It feels like we are sliding into a period of unrest, but political philosophy offers hope. *The Conversation* (https://theconversation.com), published online 29 April 2020. https://theconversation.com/coronavirus-it-feels-like-we-are-sliding-into-a-period-of-unrest-but-political-philosophy-offers-hope-137006 (accessed 31 October 2022).

Capano, G., Howlett, M., Jarvis, D. S. L., Ramesh, M., & Goyal, N. (2020). Mobilizing policy (in)capacity to fight COVID-19: Understanding variations in state responses. *Policy and Society*, *39*(3), 285–308. 10.1080/14494035.2020.1787628

Constantinou, C. S. (2022). Responses to Covid-19 as a form of 'biopower'. *International Review of Sociology*, *32*(1), 29–39. 10.1080/03906701.2021.2000069

Danish Ministry of Health. (2021). Press release, 10 September 2021. *Covid-19 kategoriseres ikke længere som samfundskritisk* [Covid-19 is no longer categorized as critical to society]. https://sum.dk/nyheder/2021/september/covid-19-kategoriseres-ikke-laengere-som-samfundskritisk- (accessed 18 January 2023).

Degerman, D., Flinders, M., & Johnson, M. T. (2020). In defence of fear: COVID-19, crises and democracy. *Critical Review of International Social and Political Philosophy* (Online, October 2020). 10.1080/13698230.2020.1834744

Dreyfus, H., & Rabinow, P. (1982). *Michel Foucault: Beyond structuralism and hermeneutics*. University of Chicago Press.

ESA, European Sociological Association. (2021). *Book of abstracts – Sociological knowledges for alternative futures*. 15th ESA Conference, 31 August to 3 September, Barcelona (online). Research Network Session 'Pandemics Politics and Policy', RN_32_T02_02, 1031–1032. https://www.europeansociology.org/publications/esa-conference-abstract-books (accessed 18 October 2022).

Esping-Andersen, G. (1990a). *The three worlds of welfare capitalism*. Princeton University Press.

Esping-Andersen, G. (1990b). The three political economies of the welfare state. *International Journal of Sociology*, *20*(3), 92–123. http://www.jstor.org/stable/20630041

Fogh Jensen, A. (2021). Epidemiernes historiske samfundsaftryk [Historical effects of epidemics on society]. In O. B. Jensen & N. C. B. Schultz (Eds.), *Det epidemiske samfund* [The epidemic society] (pp. 27–40). Hans Reitzels Forlag.

Foucault, M. (2001). *Dits et écrits, II (1976–1988)* [Spoken and written, II (1976–1988)]. Gallimard Quarto.

Foucault, M. (2007). *Security, territory, population. Lectures at the Collège de France 1977–1978*. (M. Senellart, Ed.). Picador/Palgrave Macmillan.

Foucault, M. (2010). *The birth of biopolitics. Lectures at the Collège de France 1978–1979*. Picador/Palgrave Macmillan.

Gardiner, K. (2020). *The single word that connects Denmark*. BBC. http://www.bbc.com/travel/story/20201018-samfundssind-the-single-word-that-connects-denmark?referer=https%3A%2F%2Fwww.bbc.com%2Fnews

Garland, D. (2014). What is a "history of the present"? On Foucault's genealogies and their critical preconditions. *Punishment & Society*, *16*(4), 365–384. 10.1177/1462474514541711

Gjerde, L. E. L. (2021a). From liberalism to biopolitics: Investigating the Norwegian government's two responses to COVID-19. *European Societies*, *23*(1), 262–274. 10.1080/14616696.2020.1824003

Gjerde, L. E. L. (2021b). Governing humans and "things": Power and rule in Norway during the Covid-19 pandemic. *Journal of Political Power*, *14*(3), 472–492. 10.1080/2158379X.2020.1870264

Hobbes, T. (1997[1651]). Leviathan. In R. E. Flathman & D. Johnston (Eds.), *Leviathan – Authoritative text, backgrounds, interpretations*. Norton.

Jensen, O. B., & Schultz, N. C. B. (Eds.). (2020). *Det epidemiske samfund* [The epidemic society]. Hans Reitzels Forlag.

Lindström, M. (2020). The COVID-19 pandemic and the Swedish strategy: Epidemiology and postmodernism. *SSM -Population Health*, *11*, 100643. 10.1016/j.ssmph.2020.100643

Lupton, D. (1995). *The imperative of health. Public health and the regulated body*. SAGE Publications.

Lupton, D. (2022). *COVID societies: Theorising the coronavirus crisis*. Routledge.

Lynch, R. A. (2014). The politics of health in the eighteenth century. *Foucault Studies*, *18*, 113–127.

Lynggaard, K., Dagnis Jensen, M., & Kluth, M. F. (Eds.). (2023). *Governments' responses to the Covid-19 pandemic in Europe: Navigating the perfect storm*. Palgrave Macmillan. 10.1007/978-3-031-14145-4

Maci, E., & Duboz, P. (2020). Epidémie de Covid-19 en France: Logiques biopolitiques d'un confinement [The Covid-19 epidemic in France: The biopolitical logics of a lockdown]. *Recherches et Educations*. 10.4000/rechercheseducations.8806

Macmillan, A. (2011). Michel Foucault's techniques of the self and the Christian politics of obedience. *Theory, Culture & Society*, *28*(4), 3–25. 10.1177/0263276411405348

Nygren, K. G., & Olofsson, A. (2020). Managing the Covid-19 pandemic through individual responsibility: The consequences of a world risk society and enhanced ethopolitics. *Journal of Risk Research*, *23*(7-8), 1031–1035. 10.1080/13669877.2020.1756382

Oliver, C. (2020). Of Leviathan and lockdowns. *Politico.eu*, published online on 30 April 2020. https://www.politico.eu/article/thomas-hobbesof-philosophy-coronavirus-leviathan-and-lockdowns/ (accessed 31 October, 2022).

Prime Minister's Office. (2020a). Pressemødearkiv [Press conference archives]. On the website: https://www.stm.dk/presse/pressemoedearkiv/ (last visited 31 October 2022).

Prime Minister's Office. (2020b). Pressemøde den 6. april 2020 [Press conference, 6 April 2020]. https://www.stm.dk/presse/pressemoedearkiv/pressemoede-den-6-april-2020/ (last visited 25 January 2023).

Rose, N. (2001a). The politics of life itself. *Theory, Culture and Society*, *18*(6), 1–30. 10.1177/02632760122052020

Rose, N. (2001b). Biopolitics in the twenty first century – notes for a research agenda. *Distinktion*, *3*, 25–44.

Rose, N. (2007). *The politics of life itself: Biomedicine, power, and subjectivity in the twenty-first century*. Princeton University Press.

Rose, N., & Miller, P. (1992). Political power beyond the state: Problematics of government. *The British Journal of Sociology*, *43*(2), 173–205. 10.2307/591464

Schmitt, C. (2007). *The concept of the political*. University of Chicago Press.

Sjölander-Lindqvist, A., Larsson, S., Fava, N., Gillberg, N., Marciano, C., & Cinque, S. (2020). Communicating about COVID-19 in four European countries: Similarities and differences in national discourses in Germany, Italy, Spain and Sweden. *Frontiers in Communication*, *5*, 593325. 10.3389/fcomm.2020.593325

Tønder, L. (2021). Biopolitikkens dobbelthed: Om magt og magtesløshed i det epidemiske samfund [The duality of biopolitics: On power and powerlessness in the epidemic society]. In O. B. Jensen & N. C. Schultz (Eds.), *Det epidemiske samfund* [The epidemic society] (pp. 55–68). Hans Reitzels Forlag.

Waring, J., & Latif, A. (2018). Of shepherds, sheep, and sheepdogs? Governing the adherent self through complementary and competing "pastorates". *Sociology*, *52*(5), 1069–1086. 10.1177/0038038517690680

Weber, M. (1995). *Makt og byråkrati* (2nd ed., E. Fivelsdal, Ed.). Gyldendal. (Original work published 1922)

Wiesner, C., & Harfst, P. (2022). Conceptualizing legitimacy: What to learn from the controversies related to an "essentially contested concept". *Frontiers in Political Science*, 4, 867756.

Zamora, D., & Behrent, M. C. (2016). *Foucault and neoliberalism*. Polity Press.

4 Common ethical principles and biopolitics in times of COVID-19

Jacob Dahl Rendtorff

Introduction

The COVID-19 pandemic was an important challenge for the bioethics and biolaw of health care in a global era of one world of cosmopolitan globalisation. Concern for basic ethical principles for protection of the human person in global democracy was facing the rise of totalitarian biopolitics of control of health care in many countries. Indeed, with global policies of total lockdown, strong social distancing policies, travel restrictions, and strong vaccine recommendations and restrictions on unvaccinated people, states have invented new measures to protect the social body of the state.

Therefore, it was an important challenge for the development of a sound democracy in Europe and in global society to strengthen the ethical awareness of health care decision-makers, regarding the mechanisms and principles of protection of human beings in the biopolitics of COVID-19. However, the global pandemic also raised the question of the kind of ethical principles needed to steer society through the troubled waters of the dangerous disease. The global pandemic involves questions of bioethics and biolaw (Andorno, 2013; Valdés & Rendtorff, 2022). On this basis, this chapter discusses the need and usefulness of the application of basic European ethical principles as common ethical principles for cosmopolitan ethics of the pandemic in the global community.

The theoretical foundation for this analysis is Michel Foucault's concept of biopolitics. Foucault defined biopolitics as power over the human body using different disciplinary technologies. Biopolitics is control and governance of the population, the human body, and life (Foucault, 2008). Foucault emphasises that biopolitics is political control of the population with a focus on the politics of life. In this form of biopolitics, life is what political power tries to control and govern, but the human body and life may often be on the borderline of politics and thus sometimes difficult to capture by political power technologies and disciplines. Foucault focuses on the power of the neoliberal state as biopower to govern the population. Different social discourses and regimes of knowledge such as medicine, psychology, and biology function as technologies of biopower that the government can use to

DOI: 10.4324/9781003441915-5

maintain society (Rendtorff, 2014b). Following up on Foucault's concept of biopolitics, Nikolas Rose analysed biopower and dominance over the human body through technologies of life specifically in relation to medical practice and medical technologies (Rose, 2007). In the following, we will examine the biopolitical governance of COVID-19 in this perspective with a critical focus on bioethics and biolaw.

The method of this article is a normative, theoretical philosophical method of critical analysis of different positions and conceptions in social philosophy, ethics, and bioethics in relation to biopolitics, governance of life and body, and biopower (Rendtorff, 2014a). Normative ethical analysis considers biopolitics in an ethical perspective with a focus on 'the good life with and for others in just institutions' (Ricœur, 1990). Such an analysis aims at evaluating the different normative dimensions of biopolitics of COVID-19. This can be named critical hermeneutics, following the work of the French philosopher Paul Ricœur and the German philosophers Hans-Georg Gadamer and Jürgen Habermas (Thompson, 1981). As a philosophy of social sciences, critical hermeneutics includes a methodology of interpretation for philosophy of action. Critical hermeneutics operates between power and ideology and searches for ethics through critical social philosophy (Gadamer, 1995; Ricœur, 1990).

This analysis is limited to a discussion of basic ethical principles in relation to biopolitics. There are naturally various other biopolitical perspective that could be explored regarding state strategies for lockdowns and the re-opening of society. Biopolitical governmentality studies focus on strategic government of the collective body of citizens, rather than focusing on ethical principles. The focus shifts from individual health to economic and social, technical reasoning. Nevertheless, a focus on basic ethical principles shows us that biopolitical calculations also involve policies about the ethics of individual life that have been applied to the government's responses to COVID-19.

The ethics of COVID-19 in the context of the Anthropocene

A global challenge in this context was whether the familiar basic European ethical principles of protection of human autonomy, dignity, integrity, and vulnerability were applicable worldwide as cosmopolitan ethical principles and as guidelines for concern for human beings and societies in health care during global pandemics. Indeed, these basic ethical principles were first proposed as European principles of bioethics and biolaw (Rendtorff, 2002; Rendtorff & Kemp, 2000), but since the first international seminar on biolaw in Chile in 2015, they have also been put forward as essential for cosmopolitan bioethics and biolaw (Valdés & Lecaros, 2019; Valdés & Rendtorff, 2022). Here, it is important to advance basic ethical principles for dealing with pandemics in the context of sustainability and in relation to the challenge of the Anthropocene.

We must see the rise of pandemics such as COVID-19 as a problem of the Anthropocene, where humanity as a global geological force increasingly out of control modifies its own conditions of existence with potential self-destruction as a dangerous risk (Crutzen, 2007; Grinevald, 2007, 2012; Valdés & Rendtorff, 2022). The relation between humanity and nature has turned into a warlike situation, where human beings increasingly destroy nature with pollution, e.g., the global overshoot problem where humanity uses far more resources than those generated each year or the global plastic problem where plastic pollution on an enormous scale destroys nature. Moreover, the increasing loss of biodiversity in an era of mass destruction of plants and animals is a sad expression of human dominance over nature in the Anthropocene (Crutzen, 2007; Grinevald, 2007, 2012; Rendtorff, 2019). A further challenge for sustainability in the Anthropocene is the enormous global inequality, where the people of the poor countries of the world are increasingly vulnerable to climate change, environmental destruction, and other physical and social challenges.

With these global sustainability challenges, the search for ethical principles for the protection of humanity in the global pandemic of COVID-19 in 'one world' can indeed be seen as a paradoxical consequence of the era of the Anthropocene. Here, human global power and interconnectedness also imply more vulnerability and exposure to disease with the emergence of global biopolitics and governance of sustainability as essential for the future of humanity (Crutzen, 2007; Grinevald, 2007, 2012; Rendtorff, 2019; Valdés & Rendtorff, 2022).

The challenge of the biopolitical state of exception

Critical philosophers saw this combination of biopolitics, the Anthropocene and COVID-19 as an indication of the dark side of the modern state. In spring 2020 during the outbreak of the Italian pandemic, the Italian philosopher Giorgio Agamben wrote a very critical essay about the totalitarian health policy of the attempt to deal with COVID-19 (Agamben, 2020). In his writings, Agamben can been said to follow up on Foucault's and Rose's concept of biopolitics, when he argues that with modernity 'bare life' has entered the scene of biopolitics (Agamben, 1998). Thus, we can see Agamben as a philosopher who analyses the biopolitical effort to dominate the human body as bare life with biopower and technologies of control. With this perspective, Agamben was critical of the global lockdown and the subsequent restrictions for all citizens in states worldwide. Agamben argued that the emergence of a new biopolitical state of exception in states globally was determined by the biopolitical power logic of totalitarian states (Agamben, 2020).

To protect citizens from the disease and take care of the body politics of society, states reduced the rights to life of their citizens to a 'bare naked human life' (Homo Sacer), where citizens were locked down and restricted in their basic rights to survive as living human beings. Agamben was strongly inspired by Patrick Zylberman's important book *Tempêtes microbiennes* (2013). Agamben reminds us that Zylberman with this book presents a very profound analysis of the biopolitical challenges of pandemics in modern global society. The point is that Zylberman describes how health security authorities using biopolitical calculations and security strategies become essential for international biopolitical governance. Agamben emphasises that a biopolitical security prioritisation has led to the creation of 'health terror' biopolitics based on governance following 'worst case scenarios' (Agamben, 2020; Zylberman, 2013). This logic of the worst means that global authorities such as the World Health Organization formulate scenarios involving the most dangerous impact of risk and use them as political strategies for governing a pandemic.

This kind of biopolitical governance was very present in dealing with the challenge of the destruction of humanity by COVID-19. Such a biosecurity strategy was behind the precautionary politics of governments based on total lockdown, social distancing restrictions, and strong vaccination recommendations. Following Agamben and Zylberman, this biopolitical security strategy is based on the following three important assumptions (Agamben, 2020; Zylberman, 2013):

> 1) the construction, on the basis of a possible risk, of a fictitious scenario in which data are presented in such a way as to promote behaviours that allow for governing an extreme situation; 2) the adoption of the logic of the worst as a regime of political rationality; The Leviathan of Biosecurity; 3) the total organization of the body of citizens in a way that strengthens maximum adherence to institutions of government, producing a sort of superlative good citizenship in which imposed obligations are presented as evidence of altruism and the citizen no longer has a right to health (health safety) but becomes juridically obliged to health (biosecurity).
>
> (Agamben, 2020)

Thus, there is a strong moral paradox implied in the COVID-19 pandemic. For Agamben, the disproportionate reaction of the biopolitical security policies illustrates how society will do everything to protect bare naked human life in a state of exception, leading to a perverse vicious circle of increasing state power to protect human life and restricting individual freedoms with more human insecurity as the result.

Nevertheless, there is an important problem with this strong criticism of the biopolitical security state. The paradox is that Agamben's theory also risks ending in a situation where it totally disregards the horror of the virus killing thousands of vulnerable human beings. Here, Agamben seems to demonstrate strong moral blindness of the theory of the biopolitical security state. The assumption of Agamben was that COVID-19 was no worse than the flu and that this was an example of the intensification of state power over the individual. But paradoxically, this is a good example of the moral blindness of theory, since Agamben dismisses the human suffering of COVID-19, only focusing on the biopolitical dimensions of the disease. Therefore, although reflections on biopolitical power in states of exception are important, they should not disregard the ethics of vulnerable human beings. The blind spot in Agamben's reflections was that he did not combine the biopolitical analysis with bioethics and biolaw. With his strong critique of every kind of state intervention, Agamben was in danger of ending in a damaging laissez-faire situation. But what kind of ethics of COVID-19 do we need?

Ethics and responsibility in biopolitical governance of COVID-19

First, let us examine the ethics of the different biopolitical regimes governing the COVID-19 response in different countries around the world. We can distinguish between different kinds of responses to the pandemic by different biopolitical regimes. (1) A strong biopolitical response based on the biosecurity strategy of the worst combined with *a strong bio-totalitarianism* aiming at protecting the social body of the state. (2) In contrast to this strong intervention of the biopolitical state, there was an opposite strategy which was based on a *strong laissez-faire individualism* which considered the COVID-19 as a private matter with no state responsibility. (3) Between these two extremes emerged a third strategy which can be called the *welfare state biopolitical response strategy*, based on protection of the vulnerable and weak in society following a precautionary principle, keeping in mind the biosecurity challenge of the logic of the worst.

This latter strategy can be named a bioethical response strategy that attempts to overcome the opposition between biopolitical totalitarianism and a laissez-faire strategy with no protection of individuals. The key dimensions of this bioethical response to the crisis of COVID-19 should be based on genuine concern for protection of humanity, personhood, and basic rights of citizens in society. Nevertheless, such concern for individual citizens is not possible without communitarian responsibility and solidarity between members of society. This solidarity implies concern for the vulnerable and weak as key to the biopolitical response strategy of the community (Rendtorff, 2014b). Here, we can refer to basic European ethical principles in bioethics and biolaw as essential for global bioethics and biolaw. This means that we can see the concern for the person's autonomy, dignity, integrity, and vulnerability as an integral part of a development of a humanistic ethics of medical humanities to deal with the challenges of COVID-19.

Nevertheless, developing an ethical framework for dealing with basic ethical principles presupposes the concept of ethical responsibility as essential in contemporary politics (Jonas, 2003). In relation to COVID-19, we are reminded that the concept of responsibility is important as the foundation of ethics in the fields of politics and economics in modern civilisation marked by globalisation and technological progress. Responsibility applied to welfare state biopolitics helps us to move beyond a totalitarian concept of biopolitics, since responsibility presupposes the humanistic ethics of solidarity in caring for humanity and for individual human beings. Indeed, the philosophy of the welfare state suggests responsibility for the vulnerable and weak as an essential element of welfare state policies, where the state can be seen to have an ethical responsibility that supports legal responsibility and contracts. Here, responsibility functions as a basis for the law of welfare community, as suggested by the legal scholar Mireille Delmas-Marty (Delmas-Marty, 1992).

From this point of view, responsibility is a fundamental philosophical concept that has been discussed by philosophers such as Jean-Paul Sartre (universal existential responsibility) and Hans Jonas (the imperative of responsibility) (Rendtorff, 2014a). With their concept of responsibility, we can argue that health care responsibility not only has an individual dimension of universal care for the other human being, but also a future-oriented dimension with responsibility for future human beings. The imperative of responsibility applies universal responsibility to the concern for the sustainable future of humanity; this can form a basis for the protection of the social, environmental, and economic dimensions of sustainability, as suggested by the concern for people, planet, and profit in the international ethics and law of sustainability as proposed by the United Nations (Rendtorff, 2019).

Moreover, Hans Jonas' future ethics can be related to the concept of sustainability and the sustainability challenges of the Anthropocene (Jonas, 2003). As suggested, it is important to conceive of COVID-19 in the context of the contemporary challenge to human survival on the planet. Indeed, a problem of the philosophy of modernity as proposed by modernist philosophers and scientists has been that they have forgotten the close relationship between human beings and nature. It is important that the ethics of COVID-19 reflects the humanism of responsibility in the context of protection of nature. Here, COVID-19 can be considered a strong reminder of humanity's dependence on nature since humanity was captured by the virus and was exposed to the natural forces of the disease.

Basic ethical principles as essential for pandemic ethics

Thus, with this foundation of the ethics of pandemics, we can use basic ethical principles as essential elements of responsible health care in global pandemics. Today, we need global ethical principles for protection of the human person in times of the Anthropocene, including pandemic ethics. A focus on principles is an important approach in medical ethics (Beauchamp, 2019; Beauchamp & Childress, 2019). Here, the basic ethical principles help us to develop a normative health care ethics to deal with global pandemics (Rendtorff, 2014a; Rendtorff & Kemp 2000). The basic ethical principles of autonomy, dignity, integrity, and vulnerability are proposed as essential concerns or values in providing care and protection to human beings in health care ethics and protection of patients and citizens in relation to the COVID-19 pandemic.

The basic ethical principles were developed because of a European Union Biomed-II Research Project by the Centre for Ethics and Law at the University of Copenhagen, which took place from 1995 to 1998 with 22 partners throughout Europe. The result of the research project was a scientific report to the European Union with policy proposals defining the basic ethical principles. The partners of the research project compiled the results of the project in the Barcelona Declaration, which highlighted the consensus on the basic ethical principles as European principles of bioethics and biolaw (Kemp & Rendtorff, 2009; Rendtorff, 1998; Rendtorff 2000). The principles were thus a result of hermeneutic research on the origins of the significance of the principles, based on studies of the different European traditions. As mid-level principles between metaethics and practical cases, the basic ethical principles were justified from different cultural perspectives in the different cultures and traditions in European countries. Clearly, there can be considerable disagreement on the content and definition of the basic ethical principles, requiring substantial philosophical analysis and argumentation. At the final project meeting in Barcelona in 1998, the partners agreed to the core meaning of the principles, describing it in the following way.

As a fundamental ethical principle, five important meanings of autonomy can be put forward:

> 1) Autonomy as capacity of creation of ideas and goals for life, 2) autonomy as capacity of moral insight, 'self-legislation' and privacy, 3) autonomy as capacity of decision and action with lack of outer constraints, 4) autonomy as capacity of political involvement and personal responsibility, 5) autonomy as capacity of informed consent.
>
> (Rendtorff, 2002, 2014a)

But autonomy cannot stand alone, since human beings are not always autonomous and there is a need be concerned with the intrinsic value of all human beings. Therefore, it is important to accomplish autonomy with dignity. Thus, human dignity has the following meanings as an intersubjective concept:

> 1) It expresses the intrinsic value of the human being in a community or society. 2) It includes respect for the moral agency of the human subject. 3) It means that every human being must be considered as being without price and unable to be commercialized. 4) This includes that human dignity refers to the indeterminate position of human beings in the universe.
>
> (Rendtorff, 2002, 2014a)

Nevertheless, human dignity is not the whole story of concern for the individual person. Dignity must be related to human integrity. The principle of integrity may be said to refer to the totality of life, stating that it should not be destroyed. Integrity is a coherence that in a certain sense must not be touched. This coherence is the narrative coherence of a person's life (the life story) or the narrative (historical) unity of human culture. On this basis, integrity has four meanings (Rendtorff 2002, 2014a).

> 1) Integrity as a narrative totality, wholeness, completeness. 2) Integrity as a personal sphere of self-determination. 3) Integrity as a virtue of uncorrupted character, expressing uprightness, honesty, and good character. 4) Integrity as a legal notion, where it expresses the moral coherence of the legal or medical system.
>
> (Rendtorff, 2002, 2014a)

Autonomy, dignity, and integrity are classical ideas of protection and concern for human beings that are important in ethics and human rights declarations. Nevertheless, somewhat presupposed in these ideas we can refer to the fundamental anthropological existential condition of humanity, which is that all human beings are vulnerable (Rendtorff, 2002, 2014a). Thus, a fourth ethical principle is protection of human vulnerability:

> Respect for vulnerability must find the right balance between this logic of the struggle for immortality and the finitude of the earthly presence of human suffering. As an expression of the destiny of finitude the moral receptivity of vulnerability, i.e., the disclosure of the vulnerability of the other, is the foundation of ethics in our time.
>
> (Rendtorff, 2002, 2014a)

Since the proposal of the basic ethical principles as essential for European bioethics and biolaw, these principles have been disseminated as European ethics of principles in contrast to American ethics of principles (Valdés & Lecaros, 2019). This has given them a certain legitimacy and authority as important frameworks for European health care systems, but they have also been discussed globally, including a confrontation between European and American conceptions of ethical principles in bioethics and biolaw (Valdés & Lecaros, 2019).

Thus, the basic ethical principles of autonomy, dignity, integrity, and vulnerability in the framework of responsibility and solidarity can be proposed as the foundation of a global ethics of health care in the context of a pandemic (Rendtorff, 2002, 2014a). Nevertheless, the principles are abstract ideas and core values that must be applied more specifically to the context of treatment and health care of COVID patients in hospitals. Moreover, the principles need to be considered in the perspectives of patient participation and patient-doctor interaction (Jørgensen & Rendtorff, 2018; Jørgensen et al., 2018). This also applies to treatment of patients in relation to social distancing, vaccinations, and restrictions of interactions to prevent spread of the disease.

This means that it is necessary to introduce ethical judgement as the framework of application of ethical principles as core values of health care and medical treatment of patients. In this context, ethical judgement consists of three important levels, following Paul Ricœur's theory of medical judgement. The first level is the level of prudence and practical wisdom (Ricœur, 2000). Here, an important reference point is Aristotle's ethics of prudence. This level of prudence is where the health care worker tries to achieve a pact of trust as the basis for taking care of the patient or citizen. The pact of care implies mutual trust and the promise of treatment. Applied to the biopolitical authority of health care treatment, this level implies that the authority establishes a relationship of trust and promise based on respect for the patient as a person, with the basic ethical principles of respect for autonomy, dignity, integrity, and vulnerability as essential reference points for treatment.

The second level is the level of medical deontology (Ricœur, 2000). Deontological judgement aims at universalising the precepts of the pact of care between medical personnel and patients. This is the level of Kantian morality (Arendt, 1982). The deontological character of this medical practice refers to the shared truth of the medical profession. Ricœur mentions the medical secret, but in the context of COVID-19 the deontological level refers to the ethical rules and regulations that govern the ethical decision-making of the medical profession. Here, it is important to mention the code of the medical profession and the regulations that have been developed to deal with COVID-19 by health authorities. Deontological judgement deals with the relationship between progress in medicine, e.g., the development of new vaccines and treatment methods of COVID-19, and the protection of informed consent in the pact of care. Moreover, this medical deontological judgement is very important when dealing with the relationship between the individual patient and considerations of public health (Ricœur, 2000). The biopolitical challenge to deontological judgement is to maintain respect for individual autonomy, dignity, integrity, and vulnerability while providing with public health treatment during COVID-19.

The third level of ethical judgement is the level of reflexive judgement (Ricœur, 2000). Ricœur describes this level as the level of the limits of deontology. With prudential judgement, the medical personnel move beyond deontological judgement and consider limiting situations from a reflexive point of view. In the context of COVID-19, this is the level of what is reasonable and prudent within the pact of care. This could be related to permitting exceptions to social distancing when lonely people are ill with COVID-19, or exceptions to vaccination in special circumstances based on medical reasoning. Thus, the level of reflexive judgement is the level of application of humanistic medicine in providing basic ethical treatment in the care process in a framework of responsibility and solidarity.

From ethical principles to sustainable governance of pandemics

Thus, health care treatment of patients in a global pandemic should apply basic ethical principles through reflexive judgement of the three levels of prudence, deontology, and reflection. Nevertheless, considering the Anthropocene conditions of COVID-19, it is important to consider the ethics of health care treatment in the pandemic against the background of the ethical vision of the United Nations sustainable development goals. This needs to be integrated into the triple concern for people, planet, and profit (Elkington, 1999), and should be combined with stakeholder management (Bonnafous-Boucher & Rendtorff, 2016). Indeed, the experience of COVID-19 led many countries to understand that pandemic treatment was not only a matter of close doctor-patient relationships or hospital organisation but was also linked to the global challenges of sustainable development in the different countries of the world. Accordingly, the ethics of health care, as well as bioethics and biolaw, must be related to economic issues of the practical organisation of sustainable health care, combining reflections on health care ethics with broader issues of ethics of organisation, ethical economy of health care treatment and responsible management of sustainability (Rendtorff, 2019).

This importance of integrating ethics of COVID-19 treatment in broader reflections on global sustainability can be illustrated by the discussion of the role of ethical utilitarianism or consequentialism in the biopolitics of COVID-19 treatment. In political decision-making, utilitarianism follows the principle of the greatest happiness for the greatest number. A good action is an action that provides the most happiness for the greatest number of people. Utilitarianism as consequentialism has been influential in economics, focusing on maximising welfare for poor people since such maximisation will lead to more happiness since the marginal utility and benefit of the money spent will be greater if it is spent on many poor people rather than on a few rich people. In the context of COVID-19 treatment, however, utilitarianism seemed to be applied rather conversely since a few vulnerable people who would risk dying of COVID-19 were of greater concern than many people who would not be severely affected by COVID-19.

Thus, European countries such as Denmark that imposed strict restrictions on movements in March 2020, including a lockdown and social distancing, can be said to have followed a policy of protection of human vulnerability and integrity rather than a strong traditional economic utilitarianism (Lynggaard et al., 2023, pp. 271–281). Moreover, the price of protecting a human life with the estimates of the economic costs of lockdown and support for business during lockdown was estimated to be very high compared to other treatment. Nevertheless, governments insisted on this anti-utilitarian policy, emphasising the need to protect the most vulnerable in society. Accordingly, in contrast to dominant utilitarian theory, concern for the inviolability of human life, expressed by concern for human dignity, integrity, and vulnerability, became key elements in the biopolitics of lockdown and social distancing. From this point of view, we see how concern for basic ethical principles of protection of the human individual was proposed as a core principle of bioethics and biolaw of health care behind the policy of lockdown and social distancing. Thus, protection of the fundamental human rights of the most vulnerable became a key element in justifying the strict policies of protection of individuals in COVID-19.

Nevertheless, critical voices have also insisted that the paternalist vaccine policies of many governments, strongly imposing vaccines on citizens through heavy nudging and campaigns for vaccination have elements of utilitarian reasoning, sacrificing the few who do not want to be vaccinated for the sake of the majority who can be saved by well-developed vaccination policies. But is this really a utilitarian argument? When we examine the justification for vaccination, it has strongly been emphasised that vaccination is based on social solidarity, particularly with the vulnerable and weak in society who will be better off with less risk of infection if more people are vaccinated. Thus, with respect to vaccinations, we can again argue that the basic ethical principles of respect for human autonomy, dignity, integrity, and vulnerability in a framework of responsibility were essential ethical principles for justifying the biopolitics of COVID-19.

However, the basic ethical principles in the framework of solidarity and responsibility as essential for sustainable development were also applied differently around the world. In China, a country with limited vaccination, there was a *strong biopolitical response* based on strict intervention by the authorities. The focus was on isolation, social distancing, and strong restrictions on individual behaviour to prevent the spread of the disease (He et al., 2020). This approach is at risk of being at the limits of the ethics of COVID-19, based on basic ethical principles and there is a danger of creating more vulnerability in this attempt to provide strong protection of the nakedness of bare human life.

On the contrary, the *kind of laissez-fare and libertarian* approach that at times was proposed by the authorities in countries such as the United States, United Kingdom, and Brazil, where there were few restrictions and a critical attitude to vaccinations and face masks based on distrust in the government and respect for individual freedom, can be said to prioritise the principle of autonomy at the expense of the principles of protection of human dignity, integrity, and vulnerability (Unruh et al., 2022). This approach was hard on vulnerable people in society who were exposed to greater risk of severe disease and death. However, this approach also implied fewer public costs in dealing with the disease and maybe less frustration among most citizens without high health risks who had more opportunity to live a normal life than in China, which favoured a strong biopolitical approach.

Southern European countries such as Italy, France, Spain, and Portugal can be said to have proposed a *combination of a strong biopolitical focus based on strict intervention by the authorities and a focus on ethical principles regarding the protection of vulnerable human beings*. In the early days of COVID-19 in

2020, these countries were marked by laissez-faire attitudes, but following images of many wagons transporting dead bodies out of the city of Bergamo in Italy, Southern European countries changed to a strict lockdown regime with requirements for self-isolation and social distancing to avoid the spread of the disease (Lynggaard et al., 2023, pp. 271–281). As vaccines became available, this was combined with strong recommendations of vaccination. These countries also proposed face masks in public spaces as well as strict restrictions during the first months of COVID-19 when few people were vaccinated. We can call this approach an attempt at an ethical biopolitical approach.

In Scandinavia, Sweden tried to avoid a strong lockdown in spring 2020 and was therefore seen as a country that applied a *utilitarian strategy of making a rational evaluation of consequences of actions*. However, the Swedish case was soon criticised for proposing a rather cynical response to COVID-19, where the few vulnerable and often also elderly people were sacrificed for benefit of the lives of the majority. Sweden's concept of biopolitics was also justified from a medical point of view as being based on the search for herd immunity (Lynggaard et al., 2023, pp. 257–268). Thus, the Swedish biopolitics was not justified from the point of view of laissez-faire protection of autonomy but instead based on the biological principles of creating resilience of the human species. Accordingly, medical utilitarianism was proposed as a reasonable strategy to ensure social immunity in the long run to avoid more severe damage to society. Nevertheless, the weak point of the Swedish strategy remained the fact that a higher number of people died of COVID-19 than in the other Scandinavian countries due to the less restrictive policies.

In contrast to Sweden, Denmark refused to follow the utilitarian strategy and was rather close to the southern European *biopolitics of strong restrictions, but with significant differences in the formal requirements* imposed on citizens (Jensen & Schultz, 2020). In contrast to many European governments, Denmark never introduced a state of exception with a formal legal definition, but the government appealed to the moral virtues of citizens to practice social distancing. Denmark had a strong lockdown in a state of exception where everybody had to stay at home with closed borders and only vital functions of society being allowed. This lockdown was maintained for almost two months, from 12 March to 8 May 2020. After this, there was only a small gradual reopening during the summer and autumn before a second lockdown in the winter of 2021. The arguments for the Danish lockdown were not only utilitarian; a principle of extreme precaution was combined with concern for the vulnerable and weak in society. Moreover, the justification of the Danish policy was based on a concern for maintaining the Danish welfare state. Therefore, the government provided economic support packages to all sectors of society although this was very expensive. However, the argument was that the welfare state should save lives and support its members to avoid the total breakdown of society. Indeed, we can view the Danish approach as based on a biopolitics of protection of basic ethical principles of autonomy, dignity, integrity, and vulnerability (Rendtorff, 2003). At the same time, with the concern for maintaining a strong welfare state, it can be argued that the Danish government moved from basic ethical principles to considering the ethics of COVID-19 as a matter of sustainable development with the UN sustainable development goals as the ultimate horizon of the ethical challenges of the pandemic.

Paradoxically, looking at the different countries' biopolitics in relation to COVID-19, it seems that ethics and biopolitics were integrated in the responses to COVID-19 in the sense that biopolitics and collective strategies included basic ethical principles in the design of public policies. Following Agamben, this could be interpreted as an intensified dominance of the human body through ethical principles as biopolitical technologies. This point is valid, and it is an important challenge to ensure the authenticity of the ethical response to COVID-19. However, it is difficult to deny that ethical concerns also played an important role for governments during the pandemic. Totalitarian biopolitics did not have the final word and basic ethical principles played an important role as reminders of the importance of protection of individual human beings in collective biopolitical governmentality.

Conclusion

This chapter has investigated the need for basic ethical principles for a sustainable biopolitics and ethics of COVID-19. The chapter favoured the European ethical principles of autonomy, dignity, integrity, and vulnerability in the framework of responsibility and solidarity as essential for a sustainable ethics of the welfare state. This was compared with other biopolitical strategies in the world. Indeed, the agenda of the UN sustainable development goals of action for people, planet, prosperity, and universal peace is important to remember in the context of dealing with pandemics. A core sustainable development goal is to combat and eradicate poverty. Moreover, in the global challenge of sustainable development, the effort to heal and secure the planet with a focus on global resilience also relates to the goal of improvement of the health of humanity. From the perspective of the ethics of COVID-19, the pandemic reminds us of the need to find holistic and global solutions that cover all dimensions of development including the economic, social, and environmental aspects of sustainability. Considering the COVID-19 pandemic as a matter of social and environmental sustainability, it is important to maintain the UN agenda of sustainable development when developing new programmes to deal with new pandemics on the planet. Thus, the global ethics that emerges out of COVID-19 includes maintaining an ethical vision in the management of the agenda of the UN sustainable development goals. In viewing COVID-19 as a matter of global health, it is also important to continue the programme of the green transition for people, planet, and profit on the globe. The ethical message of the sustainable development goals is that global health includes concern for the most vulnerable human beings in the process of overcoming COVID-19. Here, we can see that the focus on basic ethical principles of autonomy, dignity, integrity, and vulnerability in biolaw is essential for sustainable development. This is an important message for rethinking cosmopolitanism and utopia on the planet after COVID-19.

References

Agamben, G. (1998). *Homo sacer. Sovereign power and bare life*. Stanford University Press.

Agamben, G. (2020). *The invention of an epidemic* (Published in Italian on Quodlibet, https://www.quodlibet.it/giorgio-agamben-l-invenzione-di-un-epidemia), 26 February.

Andorno, R. (2013). *Principles of international biolaw. Seeking common ground at the intersection of bioethics and human rights*. Bruylant.

Arendt, H. (1982). *Lectures on Kant's political philosophy* (R. Beiner, Ed.). Chicago University Press.

Beauchamp, T. L. (2019). A defense of universal principles in biomedical ethics. In E. Valdés & J. A. Lecaros (Eds.), *Biolaw and policy in the twenty-first century: Building answers for new questions* (pp. 3–17). Springer.

Beauchamp, T. L., & Childress, J. F. (2019). *Principles of biomedical ethics* (8th ed.). Oxford University Press.

Bonnafous-Boucher, M., & Rendtorff, J. D. (2016). *Stakeholder theory: A model for strategic management*. Springer.

Crutzen, P. J. (2007). La géologie de l'humanité: Anthropocène [The geology of humanity: Anthropocene], *Ecologie et politique*, *34*, 143–148.

Delmas-Marty, M. (1992). *Pour un droit commun* [For common law]. Le Seuil.

Elkington, J. (1999 (1997)). *Cannibals with forks: The triple bottom line of 21st century business*. Capstone.

Foucault, M. (2008 (1976)). *The birth of biopolitics: Lectures at the Collège de France, 1978–1979*. Palgrave MacMillan.

Gadamer, H.-G. (1995). *Die Verborgenheit der Gesundheit: Aufsätze und Vorträge* [The enigma of health: The art of healing in a scientific age]. Suhrkamp Verlag.

Grinevald, J. (2007). *L'Anthropocène et la révolution thermo-industrielle* [The anthropocene and the thermo-industrial revolution]. *Ecologie et Politique*, *34*(2), 146–148.

Grinevald, J. (2012). *Le concept d'Anthropocène, son contexte historique et scientifique* [The concept of the Anthropocene: Its historical and scientific context]. *Entropia*, *12*, 22–38.

He, A. J., Shi, Y., & Liu, H. (2020). Crisis governance, Chinese style: Distinctive features of China's response to the Covid-19 pandemic. *Policy Design and Practice*, *3*(3), 242–258.

Jensen, O. B., & Schultz, N. (Eds.). (2020). *Det epidemiske samfund* [The epidemic society]. Hans Retizels forlag.

Jonas, H. (2003). *Das Prinzip Verantwortung. Versuch einer Ethik für die technologische Zivilisation* [The principle of responsibility. Towards an ethics of technological civilization]. Suhrkamp.

Jørgensen, K., & Rendtorff, J. D. (2018). Patient participation in mental health care – perspectives of healthcare professionals: An integrative review. *Scandinavian Journal of Caring Sciences*, *32*(2), 490–501. 10.1111/scs.12531

Jørgensen, K., Rendtorff J. D., & Holen, M. (2018). How patient participation is constructed in mental health care: A grounded theory study. *Scandinavian Journal of Caring Sciences 32*(4), 1359–1370.

Kemp, P., & Rendtorff, J. D. (2009). The Barcelona Declaration: Towards an integrated approach to basic ethical principles. *Synthesis Philosophica, 23*(2), 239–251.

Lynggaard, K., Dagnis Jensen, M., & Kluth, M. F. (Eds.). (2023). *Governments' responses to the Covid-19 pandemic in Europe: Navigating the perfect storm.* Palgrave Macmillan.

Rendtorff, J. D. (1998). The second international conference about bioethics and biolaw: European principles in bioethics and biolaw. *Medicine Health Care and Philosophy, 1-4*, 271–274.

Rendtorff, J. D. (2002). Basic ethical principles in European bioethics and biolaw: Autonomy, dignity, integrity and vulnerability. Towards a foundation of bioethics and biolaw. *Medicine, Health Care and Philosophy, 5*, 235–244.

Rendtorff, J. D. (2003). Bioethics in Denmark. In J. F. Peppin & M. J. Cherry (Eds.), *The annals of bioethics: Regional perspectives in bioethics* (pp. 209–224). Swets & Zeitlinger.

Rendtorff, J. D. (2014a). European perspectives. In H. A. M. J. ten Have & B. Gordijn (Eds.), *Handbook of global bioethics* (pp. 293–310). Springer.

Rendtorff, J. D. (2014b). *French philosophy and social theory: A perspective for ethics and philosophy of management.* Springer.

Rendtorff, J. D. (2019). *Philosophy of management and sustainability: Rethinking business ethics and social responsibility in sustainable development.* Emerald Group Publishing.

Rendtorff, J. D., & Kemp, P. (2000). *Basic ethical principles in European bioethics and biolaw* (Vols. 1-2). Centre for Ethics and Law & Institut Borja de Bioetica.

Ricœur, P. (1990). *Soi-même comme un autre* [Oneself as another]. Le Seuil.

Ricœur, P. (2000). Prudential judgment, deontological judgment and reflexive judgment in medical ethics. In P. Kemp, J. Rendtorff, & N. Mattsson (Eds.), *Bioethics and biolaw, Vol. I.* (pp. 15–26). Rhodos International Publishers.

Rose, N. (2007). *The politics of life itself: Biomedicine, power, and subjectivity in the twenty-first century.* Princeton University Press.

Thompson, J. B. (1981). *Critical hermeneutics: A study in the thought of Paul Ricœur and Jürgen Habermas.* Cambridge University Press.

Unruh, L., Allin, S., Marchildon, G., Burke, S., Barry, S., Siersbaek, R., Thomas, S., Rajan, S., Koval, A., Alexander, M., Merkur, S., Webb, E., & Williams, G. A. (2022). A comparison of 2020 health policy responses to the COVID-19 pandemic in Canada, Ireland, the United Kingdom and the United States of America. *Health Policy, 126*(5), 427–437.

Valdés, E., & Lecaros, J. A. (Eds.). (2019). *Biolaw and policy in the twenty-first century: Building answers for new questions.* Springer.

Valdés, E., & Rendtorff, J. D. (2022). *Biolaw, economics and sustainable governance: Addressing the challenges of a post-pandemic world.* Routledge.

Zylberman, P. (2013). *Tempêtes microbiennes* [Microbial storms]. Gallimard.

Part 2

People and everyday life

Intimacy and care when the crisis hits

5 The inclusive potentials of extraordinary life

Young disabled lives in pandemic times

Isabella Vagtholm, Hanne Warming, and Emil Falster

Introduction

> ... the COVID-19 period showed me, and perhaps also many others, how that extraordinary life isn't just a life to be afraid of, worry about and make out to be a problem from the start. It's also an exciting life, because it presents us with new ways of being, other ways of doing things. Life under COVID-19 shows how a different or abnormal existence or future isn't necessarily a problem that above all needs to be solved. Being extraordinary doesn't have to be a problem, and there are many ways to respond to and live an extraordinary life. (Thomas)

The COVID-19 pandemic has exposed and reinforced inequalities and vulnerabilities in different ways, as health in all its dimensions has been under pressure. This has also been the case for disabled children and young people, whose everyday lives and general well-being have deteriorated (Orsander et al., 2020; Shakespeare et al., 2022). Not only have many disabled people (including children and young people) been at greater risk of infection due to their reliance on different kinds of professional care services, but many are also at greater risk of hospitalisation or at worst death if infected. Due to this risk, many disabled children and young people have been more isolated and forced to live without their impairment-related services, such as physiotherapy or professional care. This absence of services is an obvious concern regarding long-term negative impacts, such as poorer functioning and/or chronic and worsening pain. Furthermore, their social isolation has been more extensive due to the risks mentioned above. Thus, they have had to do without socialising with family and friends even more than their able-bodied peers. Such extended social isolation can lead to chronic loneliness, which can have detrimental consequences for overall well-being (Heinze et al., 2021; Orsander et al., 2020).

Without neglecting or silencing the negative consequences of the pandemic for disabled people and their everyday lives, this chapter will challenge the impression that the pandemic has only had negative consequences and instead present a more ambiguous impact of COVID-19. This study examines the perspectives of physically disabled children and young people on how their

DOI: 10.4324/9781003441915-7

lives have been influenced by the pandemic. While our findings include the above-mentioned negative consequences, this chapter focuses on how the pandemic has also created new ways and spaces for participation, realising rights and promoting belonging, as these more positive experiences are prominent in our data. The aim is thus to provide a more nuanced picture.

The chapter begins with a presentation of the theoretical framework outlining the concepts of lived citizenship and the social-relational model of disability, followed by a presentation of the method used in the study and the data produced. The analysis then explores how the forced social isolation of the pandemic and the implementation of online forms of communication have created new opportunities for the participation of disabled children and young people. The focus then proceeds to how technology, disability, and stigma are intertwined and how the pandemic has affected this entanglement. Next, the analysis examines how COVID-19 did not induce life-altering consequences for these children and young people and how it triggered ambivalent emotions. This includes how they experienced a sense of togetherness and solidarity during the lockdown, as everyone had to live with barriers similar to those characterising their everyday lives. The conclusion presents the findings in the light of a concept of social crisis and points out how the insights from this chapter provide a starting point for new norms that can empower the lived citizenship of disabled children and young people.

Lived citizenship and the social-relational model of disability

Lived citizenship addresses citizenship as a contextually shaped practice and identity rather than a formal relationship to the nation-state (Lister, 2007). Thus, lived citizenship concerns the realisation of rights and responsibilities, including participation and the right to influence, and the sense of belonging and receiving recognition as an equal and valued participant in everyday communities (Warming & Fahnøe, 2017). The lived citizenship approach and Lister's (2007) values of citizenship (justice, recognition, self-determination, and solidarity) form a theoretical lens for the analysis of the impact of changes in micro-sociological dynamics to the lives of disabled children and young people during the COVID-19 crisis. Through this lens, the citizenship positioning of the children and young people is understood as a product of contextualised meaning and power (re-)producing practices through which they experience and negotiate rights, responsibilities, participation, and identity (Lister, 2007; Warming & Fahnøe, 2017). In this way, this approach focuses on the local interactional space, while acknowledging how this local space is embedded in wider complexity. Beyond the agency of the subjects involved, this complexity includes institutional and political framing, symbolic power relations, materiality, and the citizenship positions and positioning of the subjects in other spaces.

The framework combines the lived citizenship approach with Thomas' (1999) social-relational model of disability. These two theoretical lenses work well together, as the definition of disability and disablism in the social-relational model is in line with how the lived citizenship approach emphasises lived experiences. The model offers a theoretical distinction between 'barriers to doing' and 'barriers to being', the former referring to material or physical barriers (e.g. inaccessible places), whereas the latter addresses relational and emotional barriers (e.g. bullying and social exclusion) (Conners & Stalker, 2007, p. 3). Disablism affects the everyday lives of children and young people through experiences with such barriers and constitutes social oppression alongside sexism, racism, ageism, and trans- and homophobia. It is a form of oppression 'involving the social imposition of restrictions of activity on people with impairments and the socially engendered undermining of their psycho-emotional well-being' (Thomas, 1999, p. 60). Further, 'as well as enacted in person-to-person interactions, disablism may manifest itself in institutionalised and other sociostructural forms' (Thomas, 2019, p. 1040). However, disablism is not the only reason why their well-being and everyday activities are restricted. Thomas also introduces a concept of impairment effects, which are the direct impacts that impairments have on (in this case) the bodily functioning of children and young people. Impairments are bio-social and have material, bodily effects (e.g. pain, fatigue), which nonetheless are also socially constructed by medical discourses (Thomas, 2019).

Background and method

The empirical contributions have been produced as part of the work of the LIMO research centre (LIfe with a MObility [physical] disability from a child and youth perspective), funded by the Bevica Foundation and Roskilde University. A key aim of the centre is to investigate how children and young people experience everyday barriers in their lives and the resources they develop based on their experiences with these barriers. The pandemic hit halfway through a project with this very focus, which challenged the fieldwork but at the same time also enabled new (and sometimes more inclusive) methodological approaches. It also triggered a new interest in the research centre and formed the research question of this chapter: How did the pandemic affect the everyday lives of physically disabled children and young people?

Empirically, the analysis is based on qualitative contributions from 19 children and young people aged 4–25 years with different physical impairments. The contributions cover written and oral online interviews as well as essays, poems, and video diaries. The majority of the written contributions form part of a publication by a Danish cerebral palsy organisation and a foundation aimed at giving disabled young people the opportunity to share how their lives have been affected by the pandemic and the first lockdown restrictions (CP-Danmark & Elsass Fonden, 2020). Both the length and form of the contributions vary in relation to the participants' individual abilities and preferences.

The form of the interviews also varies, but they were all held online due to the pandemic, geography, and increased online accessibility. Some of the participants were recruited through their contributions in the above-mentioned publication, while others have participated in other LIMO projects and were therefore also contacted and invited to participate in this study. Some are non-speaking and were therefore interviewed in writing. These non-speaking children and young people all live together in a care home, where a teacher helped to facilitate a written group interview. The rest of the interviews were held online and were loosely structured around their everyday lives during the pandemic. The interview questions invited narratives about the changes, including positive and negative experiences, and their hopes and fears for the post-pandemic future, in an attempt to legitimise more complex and ambiguous accounts.

Disabled children and young people often find that their identity is reduced to their impairment; they are locked in the position of a deviant Other, often in terms of a medical understanding of their impairments (Falster et al., 2022; Gustavsson & Nyberg, 2015; Kittelsaa, 2014). With that in mind, for ethical and empirical reasons, questions were not asked about impairments and diagnoses, and medical terms were avoided during the interviews; instead, the interviewees decided for themselves if and when their impairments were relevant and appropriate to mention, just as they decided on their own pronouns (i.e. she/her, he/him, they/them).

The analysis of the material combines elements from narrative and thematic analysis, beginning with the analysis of each (oral or written) narrative on its own terms, asking the questions: What is at stake here? What are the key messages (plots) about the pandemic that affect the everyday life of the author/teller of the narrative? The material was then examined to identify similarities and differences in the plots and themes.

New forms of participation

A major change in the lives of children and young people during COVID-19 was the enforced social isolation, which caused school, leisure activities and other social activities to be cancelled or moved online if possible. To share their experiences of social isolation, here are two young people, Anna and Morgan, both of whom rely on different kinds of mobility aids in their everyday lives due to their impairments:

> Paradoxically, COVID and the restrictions seemed to fix one of my everyday problems: the lack of accessibility and hassles with transport. Now people became much more aware of the possibilities of online communication. (…) It was a great opportunity to take part in all kinds of things. Even things on the fourth floor. Stairs couldn't stop me taking part! I could just sit at home and be a part of it all. (Anna)

> Because it's been accessible online, I haven't had to plan so much. I don't have to plan my transport far ahead and all that. I can just sit under my duvet and watch. It's taken away some of my planning stress for going out, being sociable and doing things. (Morgan)

Both Anna and Morgan narrate how online forms of communication, as a consequence of the social isolation, actually made it easier for them to participate in social events, as material barriers that they normally experienced did not constrain them in the virtual world. They were not the only ones to have such a paradoxical experience, as Anna describes it. Several of the participants commented on how the pandemic expanded their opportunities for participation through various forms of digital platforms and virtual universes, where online communication, social meetings, and events had to take place. The reason for this experience, however, is that before COVID-19, despite formal rights of participation and inclusion and values of equality, they would normally in practice be excluded due to taken-for-granted ways of organising social life, including various forms of material barriers, such as poor accessibility for those relying on mobility aids (Falster et al., 2022). The pandemic eroded such taken-for-granted practices, and new norms emerged for responsible practices, where barriers to doing (physical interaction) became more of a general phenomenon, not merely affecting certain subgroups. When the online alternatives to physical presence became normalised, they no longer needed to be negotiated by disabled children and young people and it was no longer perceived as a 'special consideration' to include people with 'special' (and often stigmatised) needs. Morgan describes the pre-pandemic situation as follows: 'In that situation, we often used to hear arguments like: "If we allow you to work from home, then we might as well give everyone the time off!"'

Conversely, during the pandemic, online participation was generally legitimised as the only responsible way to maintain social life, work, and education. As with Anna and Morgan, this changed the lived citizenship of many children and young people from one of exclusion and a struggle to overcome barriers to one of participation and a greater realisation of their right to participate.

Online communication thereby reduced the so-called 'everyday problems' and barriers experienced, creating instead a spill-over effect in terms of new opportunities for the participation of disabled children and young people: a more inclusive space of lived citizenship, which provided greater equality.

A new sense of belonging

The two boys Malik and William also found positive aspects of the online alternatives introduced during the lockdown. They chose to contribute a YouTube video and a simple programmed game to show off the new technological skills they had developed during the pandemic. As part of the video and the game, they shared some of their thoughts on social isolation:

> I also learned to be more responsible, as I started my own esports team. When I went back to school, I felt like I'd learned a lot. (William)

> All that social isolation was fine for me, because I got my own proper laptop and I had time to start YouTubing. (Malik)

For these two boys, enforced social isolation provided new opportunities to develop hobbies and technological skills, and thus join new communities: Malik on YouTube, where he and other young people follow and watch each other's videos, and William through an esports team, where he was able to join and take responsibility for a social community. In other words, they cultivated accessible forms of communication that were legitimised during the lockdown, and thus invented new ways to communicate with peers and enhanced their sense of belonging to the new online communities.

This clearly indicates how online forms of communication could be used more in the future to include those people and groups in our society for whom in-person events and social gatherings are troublesome or sometimes even impossible, due to irremovable material barriers or impairment effects that may prevent people from moving physically and participating. This does not mean, however, that the material barriers have somehow been overcome or no longer exist or have consequences; rather, it means that practices and norms of practices matter. Due to changes in practices and practice norms, the material barriers no longer create relational barriers in the lives of disabled children and young people, and therefore do not have the same negative consequences for their lived citizenship.

The example of forms of online communication illustrates how lived citizenship can unfold in an inclusive manner through digital devices and create a feeling of participation, a sense of belonging, and greater self-determination. However, the positive consequences also indirectly reveal how the lived citizenship of disabled children and young people was restricted before COVID-19, when face-to-face interaction was the norm; possible online alternatives were not usually even considered. Consequently, this group was excluded, as their bodily reality prevented such participation. In-person interactions as the (unquestioned pre-pandemic) norm thus naturalised and individualised the exclusion problem rather than making it an issue of choice, negotiation, and critical examination in the community in question. Examples of such communities could be a group of friends, school, daycare institution, or sport and leisure clubs.

Technology and stigma

Before COVID-19, the dominant discourse among adults was that children and young people should avoid excessive screen time, regardless of whether they were playing games or interacting with peers on social media. Screen time was both a concern and reason to intervene, especially among parents. The pandemic challenged this discourse; rather than projecting an image of anti-social behaviour, online forms of communication suddenly became perceived as a means for children and young people to socialise without risk of infection, and thus as responsible social behaviour (Hansen et al., 2020). The critical voices regarding excessive screen time and the risk of isolation and anti-social behaviour related to 'hiding behind the screen' were silenced and replaced with the encouragement of, e.g., online schooling and socialising. This discursive shift made a major difference for most of the participants in our study, as online alternatives often enhanced participation in several ways (as described in the previous section). Yet this was not the only advantage children and young people found as a result of the increased and legitimated digitalisation of their lives. Online inclusion also seems to alleviate disability stigma related to physical appearance. Anna shared her experience of being stigmatised when she attempted to join social events before the pandemic: 'The wheelchair was reason enough for me to be labelled as marginalised'. In contrast, when social events take place online, her wheelchair and impairment are rendered invisible, not just giving her access to the event but also liberating her from the disability stigma related to physical appearance. While real or full emancipation from stigma might be said to remove the label of her disability based on her physical appearance, the invisibility of her difference creates a sense of not being labelled online, which enhances her lived citizenship in this context. Anna's feeling of being stigmatised by the visibility of her impairment resonates with our findings from a pre-pandemic project about the everyday life of children and young people with physical disabilities (Falster et al., 2022). Emma described the impact of the stigma she experiences when people stare at her, giving an example:

> Sometimes I understand why people look at me, but they don't have to stare. It often makes me feel like something's wrong with me, because when people stare, I'm constantly reminded that my body is different. It's so annoying.

Technologies, disabilities, and stigma are intertwined in different ways. Assistive technologies designed for disabled people tend to involve stigma, e.g. eye-tracking software or screen readers. Just as a wheelchair connotes immobility even though it actually *increases* mobility, this kind of technology enhances the disability stigma, emphasising *otherness* (Parette & Scherer, 2004). The technologies that connected us during COVID-19, e.g. for education, work, shopping, or seeing the doctor, were technologies that 'all of us' depended on, not only disabled people. Moreover, these technologies, like most technologies for able-bodied people, have not been stigmatised. Aside from Anna, many of our participants found that barriers to their equal participation were dismantled without the stigma associated with the assistive technologies. For this group, the forced digitalisation of their lives during the pandemic was emancipating, as their opportunities for participation were expanded and destigmatised. But it is also important to mention that this was not the case for all disabled children and young people, nor everyone in our study. Research on the role of digital inclusion in experiences of disability stigma is likewise equivocal and points out ambivalences (Chadwick et al., 2013; Tsatsou, 2021). In general, we may state that technologies that exclude certain groups are a common reason why some children and young people do not experience the emancipating and inclusive potential of technology. This exclusion is often because their impairment is incompatible with the technological interfaces; for instance, fine motor skills are needed to use a touchscreen. Another example is so-called web accessibility, which includes the design and coding of websites or apps that allow for the use of a screen reader. Thus, the altered practices, including increased use of certain communication technologies, which have changed the space of lived citizenship, have had positive or ambivalent consequences for the lived citizenship of some children and young people with physical disabilities, but excessively negative consequences for others.

'The only thing that has changed is the world around me'

In many countries around the world, including Denmark, the pandemic led to changes that the majority of the population found to be life-altering. 'Life is on hold' became a common figure of speech. For many disabled children and young people, however, COVID-19 had no such impact on their everyday lives; there was very little or no sense of life being 'on hold':

> Apart from my busy, sore thumbs from writing messages, things were the same for me in many ways. Everyone was on screen. Everyone had to get used to working from home and cancelled appointments. (Emily)

> In general, everyday life was almost the same as before when we got used to the new rules and measures (...) you completely forgot that daily life had changed. (Alexander, Jacob, Amelia and Elias)

Partial or total social isolation was already a part of their lives (Falster, 2021), which may be why the participants did not view the forced isolation during lockdown as a radical change. Emily stated that the only difference was that she was not alone in her inability to leave her home freely. Before the pandemic, this was the result of barriers such as a lack of suitable transport or accessibility problems at places where children and young people meet, or it could be barriers such as pain flare-ups (Falster et al., 2022). The pandemic-related barriers were more universal, as they affected everyone; in other words, when common barriers arise, the disability-related barriers do not trigger the same sense of inequality and injustice, and the space of lived citizenship moves closer to being in accordance with values of equality and justice. Some of the participants were comforted by feeling that everyone now lived under conditions similar to their own, and that they were therefore less different:

> It was reassuring, though, that there were a lot of people sitting in other places doing the same thing.' (Morgan)

While the isolation radically changed the lives of able-bodied people, our interpretation is that it created a sense and experience of togetherness for disabled children and young people, as their lives were now similar to those of everyone else. This feeling of sharing a way of living could thus create a sense of togetherness and move the space of lived citizenship towards the value of solidarity. The shared way of life during COVID-19 may provide a basis for an emergent understanding of how their different lives in 'normal' times create unequal opportunities for participation, inclusion, and a sense of belonging. It might also lead to recognition of the importance of taking responsibility for including disabled people. The pandemic could thereby have presented new opportunities for privileged, able-bodied people to acknowledge the life situation of disabled people, as the able-bodied had now experienced similar barriers. Hopefully, this might mean better conditions for disabled people to negotiate and practice their citizenship rights and identity.

The equal conditions for participation mitigated the positioning of disabled children and young people as having 'special needs' or being outside their local community. During the pandemic, they could instead participate in the same way and share (for better or for worse) the feeling of social isolation with everyone else. When the crisis changed the everyday lives of able-bodied children and young people, mostly in negative but also in ambivalent ways (Hansen et al., 2020), it reduced the perceived isolation and exclusion for many of their disabled peers. Although this in itself was positive for this group, the widespread response to isolation in mainstream society also serves as a rather unfortunate reminder of the nature of the life lived by disabled people before (and maybe also after) the pandemic.

'Your isolation ends in a few weeks – ours is for the rest of our lives'

During COVID-19, a deprivation discourse regarding able-bodied children and young people emerged and grew ever louder. Children and young people themselves expressed a longing for physical social gatherings with peers after experiencing prolonged social isolation, and adults empathised with their situation. A Danish study concluded that social isolation has created a weaker basis for a sense of belonging and overall meaningfulness in the lives of children and young people[1] (Hansen et al., 2020). While this phenomenon can also be observed among some of the disabled children and young people in our study, for those whose lives already included partial isolation and exclusion, the deprivation discourse does not resonate. Because of disablist physical barriers and impairment effects, they spend most of their time at home. Morgan explained:

> A lot of people talk about having Zoom fatigue and being exhausted. And I can understand that. But it's difficult too when it's your primary form of communication (…) Pandemic or not, I'm used to not seeing my friends for long periods of time. So I'm also afraid that when we re-open society, those of us who already have long periods where we can't be as active will be forgotten again.

Jonathan expressed similar feelings and reflections[2]: 'Your isolation ends in a few weeks – ours is for the rest of our lives.'

Although the opportunity to have the same way of life as able-bodied children and young people can create feelings of togetherness and solidarity, the able-bodied articulation of Zoom fatigue and loneliness from being unable to spend time with friends in person may also reflect their privileged position in 'normal times'. Such deprivation is the 'disabled normal', whereas it is the exception for able-bodied children; for the latter, it is legitimate to address and an object for empathy and concern among their parents, while disabled children and youth found it neither legitimate to address nor acknowledged and were not met with empathy. Experiencing this difference made some of our participants feel afraid, while some felt angry and others had both feelings. The deprivation experienced by able-bodied people can be conceptualised as relative in Davies' (1971) meaning: as a gap between expected and actual satisfaction arising from their being accustomed to better lives. The relative deprivation of the able-bodied is temporary and has a clear ending, unlike the everyday deprivation of disabled children and young people, which may be absolute deprivation. Once again, it becomes apparent how the consequences of the pandemic for able-bodied people, which they found extremely burdensome to the point of being traumatic, are actually the 'disabled normal'.

Returning to Morgan's quote, it also expresses a feeling of fear that disabled people will (once again) be forgotten and that the insights and knowledge gained from the pandemic (e.g. in relation to the inclusive potentials of online forms of communication) will not subsequently be exploited or further developed. The participants were afraid that the feeling of togetherness and solidarity would disappear and that the space of their lived citizenship would shrink when the lives of able-bodied people returned to 'normal'. This fear indicates how some disabled children and young people find that able-bodied people normally do not value and recognise them as equal fellow citizens, whose lives are also important and worth changing in a more inclusive direction; they are accustomed to being disregarded and forgotten. Although COVID-19 has had a wide range of consequences, it has also created a space for able-bodied people to gain insight into the everyday lives of disabled children and young people (as well as other groups living with similar barriers) and a more inclusive space for the lived citizenship of this group. They fear that this space (and the knowledge thereby created) will be lost when everyday life returns to normal for able-bodied people.

Lessons from the crisis

Despite certain negative effects on their lives, the COVID-19 pandemic (and thus the forced social isolation) provided new opportunities for participation and belonging for this group of children and young people. Online communication was perceived by able-bodied people as a 'Plan B', i.e. an inferior alternative to in-person social gatherings. In contrast, many of the disabled children and young people in our study experienced enhanced lived citizenship in terms of realising rights, promoting belonging and increasing participation, as every encounter and activity became an online event. Experiences of disability stigma were also reduced as their impairments and various aids and assistive technologies were rendered invisible and less limiting, which minimised their otherness. These insights form the basis for a recognition of their exclusion under 'normal' conditions and how those exclusionary social norms have been naturalised and individualised, as barriers to the lived citizenship of disabled children and young people have been neglected.

Moreover, social isolation was not as radical and life-altering for a number of these children and young people as for the able-bodied majority. Partial (and for some total) social isolation was already normalised for this group due to exclusionary and discriminating norms in addition to impairment effects (e.g. pain and fatigue). This included limited access to cultural and sports activities and socialising with peers, which was considered potentially threatening to the well-being of able-bodied children and young people but was neglected as an already existing threat for those with impairments (Falster, 2021; Falster et al., 2022). In other words, the suffering resulting from the pandemic is the norm for disabled children and young people.

A crisis is often defined as a temporary loss of balance and inability to control the forces forming the possibilities of our everyday lives. Yet this definition seems only valid for the privileged, as a crisis cannot be described as a temporary disorder or short period of change for a great number of people around the world (Vigh, 2008). As mentioned above, the changes resulting from the pandemic for able-bodied children and young people are often the norm for their disabled peers. Our study reveals how structural change (e.g. resulting from a pandemic as a social crisis) can create a space of opportunity in terms of (1) a more inclusive space for the lived citizenship of (some of) the people who used to be excluded or discriminated due to practices and practice norms (in this case, disabled children and young people); (2) insights into the everyday lives and life circumstances of disabled children and young people, and disabled people more generally. This space for opportunity can provide knowledge of differences in relation to privileges, power relations, rights, life circumstances, and exclusionary and discriminating norms for participation. This knowledge can form a basis for creating inclusion in the form of equal opportunities for participation, which will also give disabled children and young people a feeling of togetherness, solidarity, and belonging. It could be an empowering starting point for negotiating rights and responsibilities, as well as an opportunity to create awareness of how norms and structural conditions in society privilege some but exclude and discriminate against others.

Studies of how COVID-19 has changed our lives have revealed the existence of a choice between accepting the exclusion and discrimination of disabled people and striving towards equality, equity, and inclusive citizenship. A full return to pre-pandemic interaction patterns, practices, and conditions involves a return to exclusion and discrimination against disabled people. This entails a direct positioning of this group as not 'important enough' and a devaluation of the positive outcomes of their inclusion, participation, self-determination, and sense of belonging. This is exactly what many disabled children and young people fear: that the insights from the pandemic, including those regarding more inclusive forms of communication, will be forgotten and remain unexploited in the future, which basically means a full return to their pre-pandemic life situation.

However, there is an alternative. As Thomas pointed out in the introductory quote, the extraordinary life – both the one that everybody had to live during the pandemic and the one that is the 'disabled normal' – is not necessarily something to

> be afraid of, worry about and make out to be a problem from the start. It's also an exciting life, because it presents us with new ways of being, other ways of doing things. Life under COVID-19 shows how a different and abnormal existence or future isn't necessarily a problem that above all needs to be solved. Being extraordinary doesn't have to be a problem, and there are many ways to respond to and live an extraordinary life.

As our analysis demonstrates, the insights from the crisis have the potential to help us identify and critically examine the norms in our society that are exclusive and discriminating, which may also point us in specific directions in the future as to what active steps can be taken to enhance the lived citizenship of disabled children and young people.

Notes

1 The study also reveals ambiguities in terms of how the pandemic did change the everyday lives of Danish children and young people. For instance, some of the children and young people experienced less stress related to both school and their social lives (Hansen et al. 2020).

2 Jonathan's impairments cannot be categorized as 'physical', and his contribution is therefore not included in the data in this chapter. This single quote has nevertheless been included, as Jonathan so aptly articulates an experience he shares with many of the children and young people.

References

Chadwick, D. D., Wesson, C., & Fullwood, C. (2013). Internet access by people with intellectual disabilities: Inequalities and opportunities. *Future Internet*, *5*(3), 376–397.

Connors, C., & Stalker, K. (2007). Children's experiences of disability: Pointers to a social model of childhood disability. *Disability and Society*, 22(1), 19–33.

CP-Danmark & Elsass Fonden. (2020). *Livet med CP i en coronatid: En samling af oplevelser, tanker og refleksioner om livet med cerebral parese under corona-krisen* [Life with CP during COVID-19: A collection of experiences, thoughts and reflections on life with cerebral palsy during the COVID-19 crisis]. Available at: https://elsassfonden.dk/nyheder/oplevelser/alle-fortaellinger-fortjener-at-blive-hort/

Davies, J. C. (Ed.). (1971). *When men revolt and why: A reader in political violence and revolution*. Free Press.

Falster, E. S. (2021). Vi kæmper for at leve [We fight to live]. PhD dissertation, Roskilde University.

Falster, E., Vagtholm, I., & Warming, H. (2022). *Livet med bevægelshandikap: børns og unges perspektiver* [Life with mobility impairments: Perspectives of children and young people]. Akademisk Forlag.

Gustavsson, A., & Nyberg, C. (2015). 'I am different, but I'm like everyone else': The dynamics of disability identity. In R. Traustadóttir, B. Ytterhus, S. H. Egilson, & B. Berg (Eds.), *Childhood and disability in the Nordic countries: Being, becoming, belonging* (pp. 69–84). Palgrave Macmillan.

Hansen, H. R., Knage, F., Rasmussen, P., & Søndergaard, D. M. (2020). Savn, sårbarhed og socialitet blandt unge under Corona [Longings, vulnerability and sociality among young people during COVID-19]. In *Forskning i unge og corona* [Research on young people and COVID-19] (pp. 16–25). Egmont Foundation.

Heinze, N., Hussain, S. F., Castle, C. L., Godier-McBard, L. R., Kempapidis, T., & Gomes, R. S. M. (2021). The long-term impact of the COVID-19 pandemic on loneliness in people living with disability and visual impairment. *Frontiers in Public Health*, *9*, 738304.

Kittelsaa, A. M. (2014). Self-presentations and intellectual disability. *Scandinavian Journal of Disability Research*, *16*(1), 29–44. 10.1080/15017419.2012.761159

Lister, R. (2007). Inclusive citizenship: Realizing the potential. *Citizenship Studies*, *11*(1), 49–61.

Orsander, M., Mendoza, P., Burgess, M., & Arlini, S. M. (2020). *The hidden impact of COVID-19 on children and families with disabilities*. Save the Children International.

Parette, P., & Scherer, M. (2004). Assistive technology use and stigma. *Education and Training in Developmental Disabilities*, *39*(3), 217–226. http://www.jstor.org/stable/23880164

Shakespeare, T., Watson, N., Brunner, R., Cullingworth, J., Hameed, S., Scherer, N., Pearson, C., & Reichenberger, V. (2022). Disabled people in Britain and the impact of the COVID-19 pandemic. *Social Policy & Administration*, *56*(1), 103–117. 10.1111/spol.12758

Thomas, C. (1999). *Female forms: Experiencing and understanding disability*. Open University Press.

Thomas, C. (2019). Times change, but things remain the same. *Disability & Society*, *34*, 1040–1041. https://doi-org.ep.fjernadgang.kb.dk/10.1080/09687599.2019.1664074

Tsatsou, P. (2021). Is digital inclusion fighting disability stigma? Opportunities, barriers, and recommendations. *Disability & Society*, *36*(5), 702–729.

Vigh, H. (2008). Crisis and chronicity: Anthropological perspectives on continuous conflict and decline. *Ethnos: Journal of Anthropology*, *73*(1), 5–24. https://doi-org.ep.fjernadgang.kb.dk/10.1080/00141840801927509

Warming, H., & Fahnøe, K. (2017). Social work and lived citizenship. In H. Warming & K. Fahnøe (Eds.), *Lived citizenship on the edge of society. Rights, belonging, intimate life and spatiality* (pp. 1–22). Palgrave Politics of Identity and Citizenship Series. Palgrave Macmillan.

6 Ageing abjection from a COVID-19 crisis perspective

Anne Leonora Blaakilde, Karen Christensen, and Anne Liveng

Introduction

The aim of this chapter is to explore how the population of older persons was represented by the Danish government in the discourse related to the policy strategies introduced during the COVID-19 crisis from January 2020 to January 2022.

We argue that the rhetoric applied in this period and context represents a renewed contribution to the problematisation of old age as a specifically vulnerable and hence problematic phase of life, in both personal and societal terms. With the term 'problematization' we are inspired by Foucault (2003), and refer here to a global political and economic concern about the transformation related to the growth of the ageing populations in the world. This transformation has been declared as one of the most central demographic challenges worldwide since 1982, when the United Nations held the first World Assembly on Ageing (UN, 1982, 2020).

In 2021, the Danish population consisted of almost 5.9 million people, with 20.1% in the 65+ population group and 4.9% in the 80+ group (DaneAge, 2021). These two chronologically defined age categories are often applied in national policies and statistics as parameters for policy measures and distribution of welfare and rights (e.g. Danish Health Authority, 2015; Statistics Denmark, 2021).

The terminology applied in this chapter follows the Danish national discourse with its insistence on the terms 'the older population' or 'older persons' to connote persons aged 65+. The vast variation in health and life conditions for these persons is acknowledged on the main webpage of the Ministry of Social Affairs and Senior Citizens, which states:

'1.1 million people in Denmark are 65+, and their proportion will increase significantly in the years to come. Many older people are active and healthy, but a large group is also struggling with illness, degeneration and loneliness' (Ministry of Social Affairs and Senior Citizens, 2022).

Care homes and home care in Denmark fall under this ministry. About 3.6% of the population aged 65+ live in the 932 care homes around the country, and 11% receive home care in their homes (Rostgaard, 2020).

DOI: 10.4324/9781003441915-8

Furthermore, Danish policies related to ageing also include the retirement age, which is being raised with the aim of including more older persons in the labour market in the future. In 2021, the retirement age was 66.5, and by 2070 it is anticipated to be 74 for persons born after 1996 (STAR, 2020), but retirement policies are not the concern of this article.

Within this overall context, our focus is on the COVID-19 pandemic, making the older population an important target for the implementation of policy regulations. The COVID-19 crisis started in Denmark in March 2020 and lasted until January 2022, and was in political and public discourse described as consisting of three waves. These waves were related to shifts between stronger and weaker restrictions on daily life in Denmark, as the political rhetoric was the argument for the choice of restrictions (see the timeline Table 6.1).

In this chapter, we ask: How did the prime minister, Mette Frederiksen (MF), leader of the Danish Social Democratic Party and representing the Danish government, address the pandemic and its consequences with regard to the older population in Denmark? In what ways did her rhetoric enhance, or counteract, cultural values and understandings of ageing, older age and vulnerability? Which contributions did the rhetoric in her COVID-19 related speeches offer to the overall narrative of ageing and older age in Denmark? The analysis of this problematization will be informed by the gerontological perspective of 'ageing abjection'.

Research about older people, COVID-19, and vulnerability

A growing body of literature has addressed the changing conditions caused by the COVID-19 crisis and issues of old age and vulnerability have been raised, both in the Nordic context (Andersen, 2020; Andersen et al., 2021; Ó Cathaoir et al., 2021; Rostgaard, 2020), and internationally (e.g. Daly et al., 2022; Fraser et al., 2020; Ghandeharian & FitzGerald, 2022; Graham, 2022; Naughton et al., 2021; Skipper, 2021; Tronto & Fine, 2022). The literature varies in terms of perspectives and focus areas; this partly depends upon which period of the pandemic the studies are covering.

Using an ethical perspective on the pandemic as a whole, Ghandeharian and FitzGerald (2022) argue that COVID-19 has enhanced our understanding that vulnerability is an inescapable part of human life and that this reveals the inadequacy of the modern Western world's assumption of an independent actor. They suggest seeing vulnerability as a political concept, and that the ethics of care (Gilligan & Snider, 2017) can help to reorientate the fundamental understanding of vulnerability. While this represents a critical perspective on the pandemic, it also includes the potential of revealing a need to replace independency with interdependency.

Another part of the literature focuses on ageism in relation to intergenerational relations and social media (Graham, 2022; Skipper, 2021), and Fraser et al. (2020) have raised a warning related to ageism being embedded in the political responses to COVID-19, stating: 'The public discourse during COVID-19 misrepresents and devalues older adults' and 'The ageist attitudes circulating during COVID-19 make some people think that the pandemic is an older person problem' (Fraser et al., 2020, p. 692). An important contribution to this critical view comes from Naughton et al. (2021), who point out that the response to COVID-19 in the midst of the pandemic based on age advocacy represents no exception in terms of ageism. They find a well-meaning and inadvertent ageism consisting of homogeneous language, and a power binary between age and age-neutral midlife (despite the inescapable fact of higher health risks for those in midlife too) as well as a binary between abjection and glorification of older age. In other words, the twin faces of old ageism pointed out in gerontology are applicable to COVID-19 related analyses (Fraser et al., 2020). Here, this line of thought is applied in the Danish context.

In the following section, the theoretical framework of the analysis is presented.

Table 6.1 Timeline of COVID-19 response in Denmark: The timeline is constructed to show some of the most essential official responses to COVID-19 from the government and health authorities and secondarily some restrictions concerning residents in care homes

2020, January 15:	The Danish Health Authority distributes information about COVID-19 to health professionals.
2020, January 23:	Instructions are issued by the Danish Health Authority to health professionals working in hospitals.
2020, January 30:	The WHO declares COVID-19 a global emergency.
2020, March 6:	First press conference by the Danish Prime Minister, Mette Frederiksen. (PM MF) with recommendations (concerning shaking hands, travel prohibitions, etc.)
First wave:	
2020, March 11:	Second press conference (PM MF): Avoid public transport and international travel.
2020, March 11:	Lockdown. Gatherings restricted to one hundred persons.
2020, March 17:	Gatherings restricted to ten persons. Care home recommendations: no physical contact and preferably no visits. Posters stating 'You protect your loved ones best by not visiting them'.
2020, April 6:	Visits to care homes prohibited. Staff instructed to maintain distance and wear personal protective equipment (PPE). No social activities in care homes. Due to a shortage of PPE, staff and patients in hospitals had first priority to access, second priority was given to staff at care homes, and third priority to residents of care homes. Later, the situation became stabilised, as supplies were sufficient.
2020, April 24:	Visitors at care homes are allowed to visit outdoors.
2020, April 27:	Staff and residents of care homes may be tested, regardless of any symptoms. If one person (staff or resident) is infected, the care home is locked down.

(*Continued*)

Table 6.1 (Continued)

2020, May 12:	General national testing strategy for all. Visitors with PPE and negative tests allowed visits to care homes. Most activities in Denmark are quite normal again.
2020, December 16:	Second lockdown. Gatherings restricted to ten persons.
Second wave	
2020, December 27:	Vaccinations for the population with the highest priority; the oldest people.
2021, January 5:	Gatherings restricted to five persons.
2021, March:	Partial re-opening of Denmark.
2021, April:	Further re-opening.
2021, June:	50 percent of Danish population have received the first vaccination.
2021, September:	All restrictions discontinued.
2021, November:	New restrictions: PPE in the health sector.
Third wave	
2021 December 8:	Lockdown.
2022 January 26:	94 percent of the population aged 65 + have been triple vaccinated. On February 1, COVID-19 is declared a non-risk societal disease by the Danish authorities, and all restrictions are discontinued.

Ageing abjection and political speech acts

While ageing is a human condition starting from birth and continuing over the life course, later life and older age refer to the last phase of life, which has been affected during a lifetime by historical, cultural, gendered, and social contexts, and is hence saturated with huge variation and heterogeneity (Christensen & Wærness, 2021; Daatland & Biggs, 2006; Ronström, 1998). Consequentially, older age cannot be perceived as a uniform phase of life (Bakken, 2020; Gilleard & Higgs, 2010).

Studies and policies of ageing, as well as common conventions of ageing and older people, have always been immersed in an equilibrium based on a binary assessment of human capacity as either healthy or degenerated (e.g. Ronström, 1998; van Dyk, 2014). This implies a changing focus over time and contexts on either active, healthy ageing, or, by contrast, frail, vulnerable ageing. Stephen Katz has labelled the cultural approval of active bodies as 'busy bodies', indicating a busy ethics in a life course perspective (Katz, 2000), which is mirrored in the popular term *positive ageing*.[1]

Higgs and Gilleard describe this binary as a division of '… … people in later life into two classes – the fit and the frail, the agentic and the abject – a divide that overwrites other more conventional social divisions in later life' (Higgs & Gilleard, 2016, p. 63).

With their use of the concept of 'abjection', Higgs and Gilleard are inspired by the psychoanalytical work of Julia Kristeva in her book *Powers of Horror* (1982), and by Georges Bataille's essay "Abjection and Miserable Forms" (1999). For Kristeva, abjection refers to individual fear and disgust in connection with the failure to control one's body, and being unable to differentiate between being a subject and an object. In social sciences, and for Bataille, abjection is linked to social exclusion and revulsion in relation to the lower classes in society (Gilleard & Higgs, 2011, p. 136), the 'deserving' and the 'undeserving' (Higgs & Gilleard, 2016, p. 57). For both Kristeva and Bataille, abjection has the capacity to destabilise the cultural order and hence represents a threat to the dominant social order (Gilleard & Higgs, 2011). The point of Gilleard and Higgs is that, while the abject population previously was primarily characterised by poor bodies, the cultural capital of corporeal capacity at the present time has now changed to mark old bodies in frailty and vulnerability as abjects. The core of abjection is not weakness and frailty as such, but the evident failure of social intent, the inattention that betrays 'self-control' and 'self-direction'. The problem is that abjection in old age lacks individual agency, social power and corporeal ownership (Gilleard & Higgs, 2011, p. 139).

In our study of the political discourse regarding 'older persons' during risk management in relation to the COVID-19 crisis in Denmark, the term 'abjection' informs our analysis, as it focuses on attitudes and cultural values implied by vulnerability in older age.

Our approach to the rhetorical and discourse analyses of political messages is inspired by theories from sociolinguistics and narrative theory.

Speech act theory (Austin, 1962) presents a division of speech acts into three relevant categories, namely 'locutionary', 'illocutionary', and 'perlocutionary' speech acts, indicating a distinction between (1) the act of speaking itself, (2) the intention of the speaker, and (3) the consequence and/or act of what is spoken. When analysing political discourse related to the COVID-19 pandemic, these differentiations between spoken words, the presentations of restrictions and recommendations, and their consequences are very helpful. A further inspiration is the sociolinguist George Lakoff and his work on underlying values in political rhetoric; so-called *moral politics* (Lakoff, 1996). Lakoff holds that much political discourse is founded on two different sets of values which he calls 'strict father morality', and 'nurturing parent morality'. The father morality is marked by values of authority, strength, and discipline, whereas the nurturing parent morality as a value in political discourse is represented by social responsibility, respect for values of others, an ability to communicate, considerateness, and cooperativeness. These values may in some situations be intertwined and mixed, and they will inspire our analysis of the speeches by the Danish prime minister.

Data, methods, and analysis strategies

During the pandemic, the prime minister of Denmark, Mette Frederiksen (MF), held a range of press conference speeches. Between 6 March 2020 and

26 January 2022, she held 25 speeches on COVID-19 (Hansen, 2022). In 19 of these speeches, she mentioned older people and vulnerability, using words and phrases such as older persons, the elderly, the vulnerable, people at risk, grandparents, relatives, take care of each other, responsibility, and care home/nursing home. The speeches were given at press conferences for journalists in the Prime Minister's Department, emphasising the sobriety of the information based on expert recommendations, particularly by the Department of Health and the Danish Health Authority. The press conferences were transmitted simultaneously by the main television channels DR1, TV 2, TV 2 NEWS and viewed by up till 2.9 million people (Hansen, 2022), which represents a very high audience in the Danish context. The setting of these press conferences thus indicates that their aim was to make an impact on the national meta-rhetoric for understanding the COVID-19 crisis in Denmark, and on handling the course of the pandemic, which was discursively divided into three waves (see the timeline) during the two-year period. Within this wider picture of a nation's presentation and management of the COVID-19 virus, the focus in this chapter is limited to the rhetoric about vulnerability and older people, which constituted an essential part of the rhetoric of crisis (see table 6.1).

While the 19 speeches by MF cover the three waves during this period, our in-depth analysis focuses on example speeches representing each of the three waves. We assessed their typicality based on our study aim, which means that the keywords and phrases mentioned above were present in the text.

Methodologically, a combination of approaches is applied: the analysis is inspired by critical discourse analysis, regarding language as a form of social practice, representing a dialectical relationship between discourse and social structure (Fairclough, 1992). We are also inspired by Pedersen (2020), who combines Fairclough's critical discourse analysis with the actantial model (Greimas, 1987) and with positioning theory (Davies & Harré, 1990). Pedersen argues that the combination of these different analytical approaches makes it possible to create a picture of how the rhetoric relates to its context, how different parts of the rhetoric relate to each other and how the rhetoric seeks to change the surrounding world. This approach treats texts and language as able to influence what Fairclough terms the social practice, being in this sense a tool of power (Pedersen, 2020, p. 201).

In the speeches, specific categories, concepts, and discourses are identified. The choice of words is coded according to semantic equivalence: How do words and phrases point to an overall meaning? For example, a discourse of 'vulnerable people' is presented as an overall category for those understood as at risk of serious illness and death. This category connotes, e.g., older people. The actantial model is used to illustrate positions and relationships adhered to by different actants in relation to each other in the text (see Figure 6.1 for an illustration of the actantial model as part of the analysis). The interrelatedness of a variety of elements and contexts in discourses represents the quality of 'intertextuality' (Fairclough, 1992, p. 101), and this perspective is used to analyse how specific phrases like 'vulnerable people' draw on other texts and

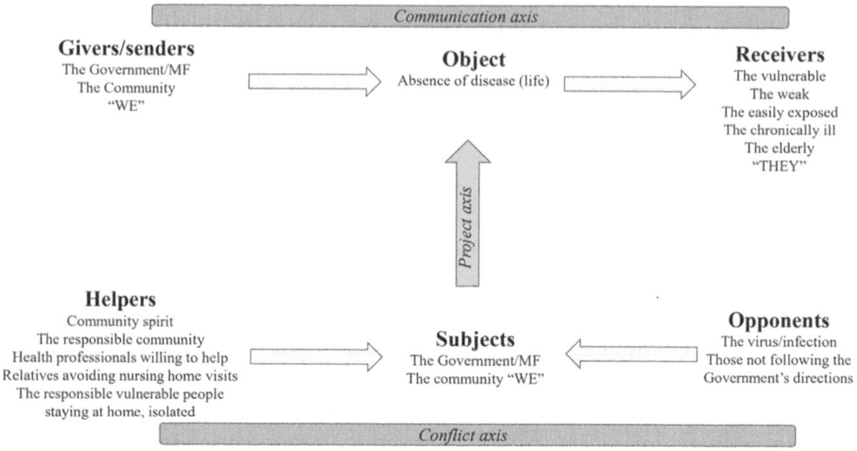

Figure 6.1 Actantial analysis of PM's first wave speech.

contexts, whereas the analysis of positioning reveals how different agents are hierarchically positioned in the speeches (Davies & Harré, 1990).

Rhetoric about vulnerability

Speech at press conference 11.03.2020 (first wave)

This speech was held at the very beginning of the first wave of the pandemic, characterised by a discourse of emergency. The objects MF introduces here are 'absence of disease', 'prevention of deaths', and 'saving lives'. The numbers of infected persons are presented along with a calculation of the speed of contagion: 'We must prevent too many from becoming infected at once. As has happened in Italy'. The axis of the project is described as an effort to avoid the spread of infection and to prevent 'older and vulnerable persons' from getting sick and eventually dying to ensure that Denmark does not end up with 'Italian conditions'. The reference to Italy is an example of intertextuality, since shocking pictures from Italian hospitals had been shown on Danish public TV channels, constituting a common frame of reference for the salience of the situation. As a subject for the project MF positions herself, the government, and the community as 'we':

> We must stand together. We must take care of each other. But in a different way than we usually do. As Danes, we tend to seek community by being close together. Now we must stand together by keeping our distance. We need community spirit.[2]

The concept of community spirit is introduced as part of the discourse about the pandemic. This spirit is presented as a specifically Danish asset, and, in terms of the actantial model, it functions as a helper in the narrative. With this discourse, MF aims to change social practices, which in this case means changing Danish citizens' behaviour during the lockdown. The community spirit refers to the responsible community helping the vulnerable citizens in society, and the term functions as an important concept in the discourse of responsibility. Health professionals who are willing to make an extraordinary effort, as well as relatives who follow the regulations of not visiting their older family members in nursing homes and hospitals exemplify the community spirit and they are also positioned as helpers. Furthermore, responsible 'older and vulnerable persons' who voluntarily isolate themselves can be seen as helpers. MF speaks directly to both relatives and vulnerable citizens, and she aligns herself strongly with the government strategy: 'Hospitals and nursing homes are encouraged to restrict visitors. With immediate effect. It is important that all relatives do respect that'. Later she adds: 'I would also strongly urge all vulnerable citizens to stay at home. Stay at home. The ones whom COVID-19 can hit especially hard'. It is indicated that staying at home is not a given.

Obviously, the primary opponent is the COVID-19 infection. The battle against the virus motivates all the imposed restrictions, which is the very reason for the speech. But those who do not follow regulations and recommendations from the government are positioned as opponents as well. At the axis of the conflict is thus the opposition between community spirit and responsibility on the one hand and the virus and irresponsible citizens on the other.

On the communication/transmission axis, the givers/senders are by and large identical to the subjects and the helpers. If Danish citizens show community spirit, meaning that they follow and respect the strategy laid out by the government, then 'we' will have the capacity to give the object, life/prevention of death, to the receivers. A discourse of vulnerability is represented by the receivers: they are positioned in a category that includes chronically ill and older people, who are framed as vulnerable, weak, and easily exposed. 'They' are the ones who will benefit from the responsibility shown by the government and community in unity, as MF states:

> I would like to emphasise again that we have a very great obligation to help especially the weakest people in our society, the most vulnerable to diseases, people with chronic diseases, cancer patients, older people. For their sake, the infection must not spread. (…) Everyone who is healthy and doesn't feel vulnerable, we have a huge responsibility for the most vulnerable people in our society.

In this way, a dichotomy is established between the category of 'we, the healthy/responsible people' and the category of 'they, vulnerable/ill/older people'. Whereas the first category of citizens is positioned as active agents ('we' can help older people by shopping, cooking, or by 'keeping an eye on them') those in the second category are suggested to be passive. The only active action 'they' can perform is self-isolation at home. In connection with the repeated references to weakness and vulnerability, and since 'they' are positioned as the target for protection, 'they' are not only presented as at risk, but also as people to be pitied. Thereby 'we' and 'they' are incorporated into a subtle, moral constellation, where 'we' function as the good saviours, while 'they' are the victims who need to be saved. In opposition to the good saviours stands the evil: the virus and the irresponsible people.

This objectification of ill, weak, and older people functions as a defence against the threat of death introduced by the virus for the healthy. If risk can be projected onto another category than the one 'we' belong to, people in the category of 'we' will have less to fear. This dynamic can be interpreted as an ageing abjection. Vulnerability, weakness, and closeness to death is placed on the shoulders of older people, keeping a recognition of vulnerability as a basic human condition at bay. Paradoxically, those who are the receivers of the object and thereby in focus for the project are at the same time excluded as speaking subjects in the discourse.

Speech at press conference 18.09.2020 (second wave)

This speech was held at the beginning of the second wave in connection with a re-introduction of restrictions and is strongly marked by a discourse of seriousness and a discourse of responsibility. The objects introduced by MF in this speech are a delay in the increase of infection and an avoidance of a total shutdown of society. She begins with an appraisal of Denmark's positive situation compared to spring 2020, because of the highest testing rate in the world. Through an intertextual reference to awful situations shown in the news, the Danish situation is compared to that in other European countries, which is described as much worse. Then MF turns to the numbers of infected citizens and calculations of the speed of contagion. The COVID-19 strategy introduced by the government is depicted as a fight against the disease. The project axis describes an effort to delay the increase in the number of infected persons, an argument for the necessity of new restrictions, and an appeal to the sense of responsibility of health professionals, of young people, and of the community, which should enable the objects to be reached.

As the subject for the project MF positions herself, the government, and the responsible community as 'we'.

> ... until we get a vaccine or a very, very effective treatment, our super weapons are still what we do individually and together, and therefore we will still have to stand together in Denmark by keeping our distance and all of us showing the necessary community spirit.

Seen through the lens of the actantial model, the Danish testing strategy, detection of infection chains, and the established possibility of self-isolation, all introduced by the government, function as helpers. In addition, the population functions as a helper when citizens adhere to governmental restrictions and recommendations; they avoid social contact, isolate themselves if infected, and show community spirit.

The infection and the infection chains are positioned as opponents. Young people, who are claimed not to show the required responsibility and thus add risk to the incentive to break the infection chains, also function as opponents. MF agrees with this assertion:

> And the situation is still, and I can hardly say this urgently enough, that a young person can pass on – give COVID-19 to an older or other vulnerable person, who in the worst case may die from the virus.

At the conflict axis, the Danish COVID-19 strategy (testing and isolation), community spirit, and responsible behaviour are therefore in opposition to the virus and to irresponsible citizens, especially young ones. According to the quote, they can end up being responsible for the death of older people. As seen earlier, the responsibility discourse turns into a moral discourse, where it is easily detected who are morally correct, and who are not. Even though young people are now warned that the virus can also be a threat for them, the victims of the alleged irresponsibility are still claimed to be the older and vulnerable people, but those who are expected to care for them are also included in the at-risk category: 'Unfortunately, we see more infected people among our health staff in hospitals and among the most vulnerable, for example, in nursing homes, and this is obviously serious'.

On the communication axis the givers are, as seen in the analysis of the first speech, by and large identical with the subjects and helpers. The government, the community spirit, and in the future the vaccines are positioned as givers. If 'we' follow government restrictions and advice, 'we' can give the object (delay of infection increase and avoidance of a total shutdown of society) to the receivers. The category of receivers is far broader than during the first wave. It includes the population, both young and old, vulnerable people, older people, and nursing home residents, who constitute the 'they', in addition to the Danish economy and Danish business.

Compared to the rhetoric during the first wave, it is notable that who/what are considered at risk, if 'we' do not follow the government strategy, is far more comprehensive. Not only are vulnerable and older people at risk, but the risk now includes everyone in society as well as the Danish economy and business. However, older and vulnerable people still form a homogeneous group in society who are not assigned any agency in the fight against COVID-19.

Speech at press conference 08.11.2021 (third wave)

While responsibility was part of the discourse in both the first and second waves, it comes to the forefront in the third wave. Representing the third wave, this speech carries a strong discourse of responsibility and morals, this time in relation to vaccines. The speech addresses an object of an open society where everybody is vaccinated. MF introduces this object by pointing out two sides of the situation in this third wave. On the one hand, she presents Denmark as having reached a relatively high degree of control compared to the situation under the second wave. In this sense, the situation under the second wave with much less control represents the intertextual importance at this third stage. On the other hand, she describes the situation as very serious, and 'in some ways as more worrying than under the prior epidemic waves', referring particularly to the pressure on the hospital sector, if too many people need to be admitted. The subjects who will do whatever needs to be done to reach the object of an open society comprise 'we', including MF and the nation of Denmark, but also the community in Denmark: '*That* responsibility we have towards each other and society in general to avoid a breakdown of the health services – yes, that still applies'. Thus, the project axis forms an appeal to all those who are willing to contribute to achieve the open society. But there is more to learn from the speech as a powerful speech action.

The discourse in this speech of the third wave divides the population of Denmark into two categories: those who have agreed to be vaccinated and those who have not. Therefore, the communication axis from the sender, the government of Denmark and MF, regarding the object of an open society, goes to the receivers of the message: all residents in Denmark (vaccinated or not vaccinated), and particularly addresses the latter group, but also other groups who can help (such as health personnel, see below). The discourse operating in this speech is, as previously seen, one of responsibility. This responsibility implies a much more serious division of people in Denmark than just between vaccinated/unvaccinated persons, because this discourse demarcates a group of people who are responsible towards the most vulnerable groups in Denmark (older people), who therefore actively accept the offer of vaccination in contrast to those who do not. As MF needs to take account of the fact that nobody can be forced to be vaccinated, and everyone must make her/his own decision, the unvaccinated people are only called '... those who are not vaccinated'. The discourse of responsibility, however, places them in the category of passive, irresponsible people who do not represent goodwill. The unvaccinated represent 12% of those offered vaccination, and they are 'punished' by the government and the prime minister by exclusion from the 'we': 'We have impressively strong support for vaccination in Denmark compared to foreign countries. But this is not enough, and we need more to join us. We need to get the last group involved now'. Drawing upon the intertextual feature of foreign countries, Denmark can reach the highest level by involving the last (irresponsible) group to become part of the Danish community, the 'we'.

There is, however, another important actor related to the responsibility discourse placed on the conflict axis, namely health personnel. They can either be helpers, by putting in an extra effort, despite already '... rushing around the hospital wards', and MF (as she stated herself) being aware of their frustration regarding low pay and poor working conditions, or they can be opponents by not being willing to 'go the extra mile', thus not helping to avoid more virus infection in Denmark.

While the speech and its appeals are all about the protection of 'the most vulnerable in our society', this group is abjected by playing the role of the invisible third party, without any say, any voice and any differentiation including for example their own choice between being vaccinated or not. Old age is abjected through homogenisation that ignores all forms of heterogeneity in old age and by depriving them of their agency; they are reduced to representing only vulnerable people at risk of infection. The vaccination battle between helpers and opponents at the conflict axis takes place without their involvement. In this way older age is transformed into one group, the at-risk group, and their situation is presented as the outcome of the we-group conflict, which they are not part of.

Concluding discussion

The concluding discussion consists of two parts. The first part is based on the analysed speeches by MF comprising elements of both discursive and social practice in Fairclough's sense. While we draw conclusions about the discursive and rhetorical findings from the speeches, they can also be related to social practice in terms of changes in restrictions in the three waves, based on the timeline overview. In the second part, we discuss the findings in relation to earlier research contributions.

MF's speeches about COVID-19, divided into three waves, in 25 press conferences in 2020–2022 can be characterised as locutionary speech acts in terms of Austin's concepts in his speech act theory (Austin, 1962). In that sense, the speeches 'only' consist of words. However, these speeches imply political intentions as well as effects for people in real life, which Austin terms illocutionary and perlocutionary speech acts, respectively. The illocutionary speech acts include the political intentions to manage the pandemic of COVID-19 and involve an underlying moral discourse about human vulnerability and societal responsibilities and obligations. When analysed in this sense, the speeches combine illocutionary and perlocutionary speech acts, as they reveal underlying rationalities as well as representing actions with consequences for people's lives caused by the locutionary and illocutionary speech acts. Thus, what kinds of illocutionary and perlocutionary speech acts are found here? A comparison of the three parts reveals that, as an illocutionary speech act, ageing abjection is present in all three speeches. In the first speech, older persons are positioned with vulnerable and ill citizens in one homogeneous category, comprising citizens at risk. In the second speech, this homogeneous group is still positioned as being at risk, but these citizens are no longer the only ones in focus for the project initiated by MF and the government. During the second wave the focus is broadened to include most of the Danish population as well as the Danish economy and business. Older persons are not ascribed any agency in the first wave, but are positioned as passive receivers of the object provided by the community, if they behave responsibly. The example speech from the second wave establishes an antagonistic position between younger and older people. Younger people are positioned as opponents through their irresponsible behaviour, while older people are presented as the potential victims of this behaviour. The consequences of this speech, as a perlocutionary speech act, particularly from the first wave, but also from the second wave, involve isolation from the rest of society, especially for people living in care homes, but also including younger people. This consequence of isolation of older persons was commented on and criticised, by, e.g., the Danish organisation DaneAge, which expressed concern for the 41 000 inhabitants of Danish care homes, and for those who were isolated in their homes and receiving less home care than under normal circumstances (DaneAge, 2021), which further reduced their contact with the outside world.

In the illocutionary speech act as presented during the third wave, older persons are construed as belonging to a single homogenised vulnerable group, invisible as active subjects. The discourse of responsibility is strongly emphasised and increasingly connected to a moral discourse. Now the responsibility discourse covers the issue of accepting the vaccine: the vaccinated are unambiguously positioned as good, while the unvaccinated represent evil. The struggle between helpers and opponents is framed as a moral question, in which there is no doubt what the morally right thing is to do. Where the dichotomies between helpers and opponents are morally emphasised in the first and second speeches, morals are pivotal in the third speech. In this sense, a development can be traced in MF's speeches, as she first positions herself and the government through a discourse of nurturing parent morality implying empathy, helping each other, providing equality and societal responsibility, then re-positions herself through a discourse of strict father morality comprising strength, authority, and values of moral health, representing a logic of disease connected to immoral people who may be dangerous, because their immorality may spread (Lakoff, 1996, pp. 101, 137). During the first and second waves the lockdowns induced loneliness and social isolation, which called for attention. There was a significant concern about the risk of loneliness. As an incentive to counteract the loneliness, national funding was established to provide social support to the vulnerable persons in question.[3] When the third wave arrived, the social practice which was intended by the perlocutionary speech act was far more nuanced than earlier in the pandemic. Whereas the Danish population during the first and second waves seemed struck by fear, further criticism of the strict lockdown emerged at the time of the third wave. MF's drawing on a strict father morality can be understood in this connection; strength and authority must now be employed in a more direct manner. The criticism concerned the general isolation of the older population, not only those living in care homes. These examples make it clear that the locutionary speech acts by MF during the pandemic included perlocutionary acts of real-life consequences for the social and mental life of many citizens, including people in the older population.

The positioning of older and vulnerable persons in one homogenous group during the three waves exemplifies old age as abjection, which, following Gilleard and Higgs (2011), represents an unconscious, social notion which may contain collective anxieties of weakness, decay, and lack of bodily control. This projection of aspects of the common human condition into an invisible 'black box' relieves people who identify with earlier life stages from recognising their own vulnerability. Especially during the first wave, this psychological dynamic is activated by the political speeches. Furthermore, Higgs and Gilleard state that what happens when a person is willing to act responsibly towards abjection in order to change the abject status of another, the agency of the person to whom help is given is effectively constrained, while agency is enhanced in the giver (Higgs & Gilleard, 2016, p. 64). In this case, agency is enhanced in politicians and younger population groups who also act responsibly. Especially the prime minister, MF, is represented with parental morals as a helper whose initiatives may prevent danger, but also remove agency from the group of abjects. 'The person's impotence to "unfrail" themselves, to recover or restore his or her state as an agent, then renders the person doubly abject, having become "irretrievably" frail' (Higgs & Gilleard, 2016, p. 64).

In the European context, where Denmark scored high on control of the virus and had a relatively fast response to the pandemic, limiting the number of COVID-19 related deaths (Daly et al., 2022), it may be surprising that our analysis so clearly indicates the abjection of older persons, thus confirming the statement by Fraser et al. (2020) about saturating ageism in the political response to the pandemic. However, this paradox of ageism in a Nordic welfare state that aims at equality along a range of dimensions such as age may be interpreted in the same way as pointed out by Naughton et al. (2021): the social democratic policies may correspond to their findings regarding a kind of well-meaning ageism by age advocacy representatives. Particularly within the discourse of seriousness under the second wave, it was stressed that Denmark was like a community where everyone stuck together and took care of each other (here focusing on the younger people who should be caring about the older people in the community). Can we then infer from this, that the political rhetoric is in a positive way revealing and supporting an interdependent perspective on the vulnerability of human life, as suggested by, e.g., Ghandeharian and FitzGerald (2022), especially concerning intergenerational dependency and solidarity? To some extent, we may confirm this. However, we must reject this conclusion, since the interdependent discourse is one-sided, moving simply from 'helpers' to those who need help, and biased by construing the receivers as a homogeneous group of helpless older persons. We therefore agree with the suggestion of the relevance of a more fundamental relational approach, which also includes the importance of context, such as the ethics of care (Gilligan & Snider, 2017). As the ethics of care implies a vital respect for the individual in relation to the caregiver, it may also help to prevent the way that rhetorical politics, when implemented in practice, including nursing homes and people's own homes, would result in violation of the right to health (Ó Cathaoir et al., 2021).

Notes

1 We encourage the reader to search for this term on the world wide web.
2 This is our translation of the Danish term "samfundssind", which can also be translated as social-mindedness.
3 An example of such incentives from the government was a fund provided by the Ministry of Culture in spring 2020 for activities to create social substitutions for the isolation. The Ministry described the target group as 'vulnerable, marginalised and older people' (Ministry of Culture Denmark, 2020).

References

Andersen, J. G. (2020). Corona-epidemi og corona-politik i Danmark og andre lande – en uventet konvergens? [The COVID-19 pandemic and COVID-19 politics in Denmark and other countries: An unexpected convergence?]. *SOC DOK*, *2*(1), 4–13. http://www.socdok.dk/SOC%20DOK%20%202.aarg.%20nr.%201.pdf

Andersen, P. B., Høeg, A. L. T. N., Christensen, H. R., Jacobsen, B. A., Kühle, L., & la Cour, P. (2021). Befolkningens reaktion på COVID-19 set i lyset af aviser og andre medier [The population's reaction to COVID-19 in the light of newspapers and other media]. *Religionsvidenskabeligt Tidsskrift*, *72*, 19–41.

Austin, J. (1962/1975). *How to do things with words*. Oxford University Press.

Bakken, R. (2020). *Alle vil leve lenge, men ingen vil bli gamle* [Everybody wants to live a long life, but nobody wants to become old]. Fagbokforlaget.

Bataille, G. (1999). Abjection and miserable forms. In S. Lotringer (Ed.), *More and Less* (pp. 8–13). MIT Press.

Christensen, K., & Wærness, K. (2021). Alderdom og ulikhet [Old age and inequality]. In S. Grønmo, A. Nilsen, & K. Christensen (Eds.), *Ulikhet: Sosiologiske perspektiver og analyser* [Inequality: Sociological perspectives and analyses] (pp. 197–219). Fagbokforlaget.

Daatland, S., & Biggs, S. (Eds.) (2006). *Ageing and diversity: Multiple pathways and cultural migrations*. Policy Press.

Daly, M., León, M., Pfau-Effinger, B., Ranci, C., & Rostgaard, T. (2022). COVID-19 and policies for care homes in the first wave of the pandemic in European welfare states: Too little, too late? *Journal of European Social Policy*, *32*(1), 48–59. 10.1177/09589287211055672

DaneAge (Ældresagen). (2020). *Isolationen af svage ældre går for vidt* [The isolation of vulnerable elderly people is going too far]. https://www.kristeligt-dagblad.dk/danmark/aeldre-sagen-isolationen-af-svage-aeldre-gaar-vidt

DaneAge. (2021). *Ældre i tal. Befolkning og fremtid - 2021*. [Older people in figures. The population and the future – 2021]. Retrieved April 8, 2022, from https://www.aeldresagen.dk/presse/viden-om-aeldre/aeldre-i-tal/2021-befolkning-og-fremtid

Danish Health Authority. (2015). *Håndbog i rehabiliteringsforløb på ældreområdet efter lov om social service* [Handbook of rehabilitation for older people based on the Social Services Act]. Retrieved April 8, 2023, from https://www.sst.dk/da/nyheder/2016/~/media/6D27215F08464CA0A68E949BBA4BD23B.ashx

Davies, B., & Harré, R. (1990). Positioning: The discursive production of selves. *Journal for the Theory of Social Behaviour*, *20*(1), 43–63.

Fairclough, N. (1992). *Discourse and social change*. Polity Press.

Foucault, M. (2003). *Madness and civilization*. Routledge.

Fraser, S., Lagacé, M., Bongué, B., Ndeye, N., Guyot, J., Bechard, L., Garcia, L., Taler, V., Adam, S., Baaulieu, M. Bergeron, C., Boudjemadi, V., Desmette, D., Donizzetti, A.R., Éthier, S., Garon, S., Gillis, M., Levasseur, M., ... Tougas, F.; CCNA Social Inclusion and Stigma Working Group. (2020). Ageism and COVID-19: What does our society's response say about us? *Age and Ageing*, *49*(5), 692–695. 10.1093/ageing/afaa097

Ghandeharian, S., & FitzGerald, M. (2022). COVID-19, the trauma of the 'real' and the political import of vulnerability. *International Journal of Care and Caring*, *6*(1-2), 33–47. https://doi-org.ep.fjernadgang.kb.dk/10.1332/239788221X16190193887799

Gilleard, C., & Higgs, P. (2010). Aging without agency: Theorizing the fourth age. *Ageing & Mental Health*, *4*(2), 121–128. 10.1080/13607860903228762

Gilleard, C., & Higgs, P. (2011). Ageing abjection and embodiment in the fourth age. *Journal of Aging Studies*, *25*(2), 135–142. 10.1016/j.jaging.2010.08.018

Gilligan, C., & Snider, N. (2017). The loss of pleasure, or why we are still talking about Oedipus. *Contemporary Psychoanalysis*, *53*(2), 173–195. https://doi-org.ep.fjernadgang.kb.dk/10.1080/00107530.2017.1310586

Graham, M. E. (2022). "Remember this picture when you take more than you need": Constructing morality through instrumental ageism in COVID-19 memes on social media. *Journal of Aging Studies*, *61*. 10.1016/j.jaging.2022.101024.

Greimas, A. J. (1987). Actants, actors, and figures. In A. J. Greimas (Ed.), *On meaning: Selected writings in semiotic theory* (pp. 106–120). University of Minnesota Press.

Hansen, M. (2022, January 28). Slut med coronapressemøder med seertal, de fleste kun kan drømme om [The end of COVID-19 press conferences with numbers of viewers most people can only dream of]. *TV2 Kommunikation* (Communication). https://omtv2.tv2.dk/nyheder/2022/01/slut-med-coronapressemoeder-med-seertal-de-fleste-kun-kan-droemme-om/

Higgs, P., & Gilleard, C. (2016). *Personhood, identity and care in advanced old age*. Bristol University Press.

Katz, S. (2000). Busy bodies: Activity, aging and the management of everyday life. *Journal of Aging Studies*, *14*(2), 135–152.

Kristeva, J. (1982). *Powers of horror: An essay on abjection*. Columbia University.

Lakoff, G. (1996). *Moral politics. What conservatives know that liberals don´t*. University of Chicago Press.

Ministry of Culture Denmark. (2020, June 20). *Kultur og foreningsaktiviteter hjælper sårbare, udsatte og ældre under corona-krisen* [Culture and community activities help the vulnerable, the marginalized and the elderly during the COVID-19 crisis]. https://slks.dk/nyheder/2020/tilskud/kultur-og-foreningsaktiviteter-hjaelper-saarbare-udsatte-og-aeldre-under-corona-krisen

Ministry of Social Affairs and Senior Citizens. (2022). *Ældreområdet. Om arbejdsområdet* [Working with older people]. Retrieved April 2, 2022, from https://sm.dk/arbejdsomraader/aeldreomraadet

Naughton, L., Padeiro, M., & Santana, P. (2021). The twin faces of ageism, glorification and abjection: A content analysis of age advocacy in the midst of the COVID-19 pandemic. *Journal of Aging Studies*, *57*. 10.1016/j.jaging.2021.100938

Ó Cathaoir, K., Gunnarsdóttir, H. D., Aasen, H., Kimmel, K.-M., Lohiniva-Kerkelä, M., Rognlien, I. G., & Westerhäll, L. V. (2021). Older persons and the right to health in the Nordics during COVID-19. *European Journal of Health Law*, *28*(5), 417–444.

Pedersen, K. (2020). Diskursanalyse i politisk kommunikation [Discourse analysis in political communication]. In N. M. Nielsen & K. Pedersen (Eds.), *Politisk kommunikation i humanistisk perspektiv* [Political communication in a humanistic perspective] (pp. 199–216). Djøf Forlag.

Ronström, O. (1998). Pigga pensionärer och populärkultur [Active seniors and popular culture]. In O. Ronström (Ed.), *Pigga pensionärer och populärkultur* [Active seniors and popular culture] (pp. 9–47). Carlssons.

Rostgaard, T. (2020). The COVID-19 long-term care situation in Denmark. *LTCcovid, International Long-Term Care Policy Network, CPEC-LSE.* https://ltccovid.org/wp-content/uploads/2020/05/The-COVID-19-Long-Term-Care-situation-in-Denmark-29-May-2020.pdf

Skipper, A., & Rose, D. J. (2021). #BoomerRemover: COVID-19, ageism, and the intergenerational twitter response. *Journal of Aging Studies*, *57*. 10.1016/j.jaging.2021.100929

STAR. (2020). *Folkepension nu og fremover* [The state pension now and in the future]. Styrelsen for Arbejdsmarked og Rekruttering/The Danish Agency for Labour Market and Recruitment. Retrieved April 2, 2022, from https://star.dk/ydelser/pension-og-efterloen/folkepension-tidlig-pension-foertidspension-og-seniorpension/folkepension/folkepensionsalderen-nu-og-fremover/

Statistics Denmark (2021). *Ældres helbred og brug af sundhedsydelser* [Older people's health and use of health services]. Retrieved April 8, 2022, from https://www.dst.dk/da/informationsservice/blog/2021/11/aeldre

Tronto, J., & Fine, M. (2022). 'Long COVID' and seeing in the pandemic dark. Editorial, Special Issue: Care, caring and the global COVID-19 pandemic. *International Journal of Care and Caring*, 6(1-2), 3–12. https://doi-org.ep.fjernadgang.kb.dk/10.1332/239788221X16383754538816

UN. (1982). *Report of the World Assembly on Ageing*. Vienna, 26 July to 6 August. UN Publication. Retrieved April 8, 2022, from https://www.un.org/esa/socdev/ageing/documents/Resources/VIPEE-English.pdf

UN. (2020). *Global Issues. Ageing*. Retrieved April 8, 2022, from https://www.un.org/en/global-issues/ageing

van Dyk, S. (2014). The appraisal of difference: Critical gerontology and the active-ageing paradigm. *Journal of Ageing Studies*, *31*, 93–103. 10.1016/j.jaging.2014.08.008

7 Challenges to relationship intimacy during COVID-19

LATT (living apart together transnationally couples)

Rashmi Singla, Aruna Jha, and Christina Naike Runciman

Introduction

Couples living apart together (LAT) are increasing, but this is an understudied category of intimate couple relationships. LAT couples increasingly challenge the axiom 'intimate couples stay under the same roof.' In this chapter, we present the LATT (living apart together transnationally) couple, where the partners live in two different countries (Singla & Varma, 2019). External factors such as restrictive immigration policies and suspicion about motives for migration affect the mental health and well-being of LATT couples (Holmes, 2014), while gendered expectations challenge the relationship between the partners.

The World Health Organization has reported that the COVID-19 pandemic, which started in January 2020, is now (2023) over in most of the world. However, the COVID-19 agenda took over many peoples' lives in 2020–2021. The LATT couples presented in this chapter lived on different continents. Not knowing when they would be together again affected the mental health and well-being of LATT partners during extensive worldwide lockdowns that prevented travel and curtailed residence abroad. This chapter focuses on how two couples faced this sudden situation, their strategies for coping with externally imposed travel and immigration restrictions, and their relationship maintenance process.

The following sections describe seminal studies on couples dealing with intimacy and distance while highlighting major theoretical concepts that apply to LATT couples. The chapter presents our empirical study methodology, including ethical considerations and data analysis strategies. From the overall thematic analysis, two overarching themes (1) maintaining intimate relationships despite distance and (2) the impact of the pandemic are highlighted through the two case studies. The chapter concludes with a discussion of policy implications and recommended psychosocial interventions.

Background

LAT: New forms of cohabitation in couples

Recent decades have seen a steady increase in intimate couples who do not follow the traditional, conventional understanding of cohabitation as living

DOI: 10.4324/9781003441915-9

under one roof. LAT couples manage the coexistence of geographical distance and emotional intimacy for a variety of reasons, including employment, education, immigration regimes, and particular emotional dynamics. The distance between the two partners' homes may vary from the next block, a nearby neighbourhood, the same metropolitan area (Kobayashi et al., 2017), a different city in the same country (Holmes, 2014), to different countries (Stafford, 2005). LATT couples is a recently coined term for multi-local couples (Beck & Beck-Gernsheim, 2013), where intimate partners live apart in different countries while maintaining two jobs and homes.

Four decades of international research on LAT couples highlight specific aspects of their situation. Regarded as 'dual residence, dual career couples', LAT couples represent a new pattern of couple relationships (Gerstel & Gross, 1984). This dual residence pattern differs from the traditional pattern of husbands leaving home for work for limited periods or, more recently, wives leaving the Global South (Parrenas, 2005). While work is an important source of identity and satisfaction for the couple (Lindemann, 2019; Reutschke, 2010), how work and the couple's relationship are balanced is a major concern (Carter et al., 2016). Scholars highlight the importance of relationships (Holmes, 2014), while a gendered bias challenges female autonomy even for privileged professional women, especially in view of the 'trailing spouse phenomenon' (Grover & Schliewe, 2020). Couples acknowledge the advantages and disadvantages of living apart together, citing the additional effort needed to maintain intimacy across distance, difficulty in maintaining a sense of order while being together, and elevated expectations for reunions. The above-mentioned authors make little mention of couples living in different countries who have additional challenges related to *immigration policies, reunion across national borders,* and *time zone differences*, which are covered in this chapter.

During COVID-19, people reported a variety of problems, including concerns for individual health and well-being, subsyndromal mental health problems, challenges to personal relationships, loss of future time perspective, adaptation to changes, and the reactions of society, government, and the media (Rajkumar, 2020). An international study on same-sex couples found that the perceived COVID-19 threat negatively predicted relationship satisfaction (Li & Samp, 2021). Being able to plan future dates for physical intimacy is a vital coping mechanism for partners in long-distance relationships. During COVID-19, increased travel restrictions and quarantine rules between countries affected these couples' usual ways of handling and coping with their LATT relationship (Abrahamson, 2021). On the other hand, *relational well-being* mitigated any increases in individual distress after COVID-19 restrictions were introduced (Rajkumar, 2020) and brought forth new perspectives on how LATT couples maintained their relationships while facing the challenges of COVID-19.

Exploring the couples

The theoretical framework

This research uses an eclectic theoretical framework that includes Valsiner's (2014) cultural psychology perspective focusing on personal agency and social-cultural-historical contexts. In psychology, eclecticism is one of the key conditions for conducting scientific research (Køppe, 2012). An eclectic theoretical framework combining different theoretical perspectives enhances our ability to grasp the complexity of the subject under analysis. Our framework also draws on Holmes' model for understanding distance relationships as a form of contemporary intimacy, comprising four significant elements: diversity, complex situatedness, embodied relationality, and emotional reflexivity (Holmes, 2014; 2019). The first two elements emphasise the differences and the specific contexts in the analysis of the two cases. While embodied relationality directs our attention towards the physical dimension in relationships, emotional reflexivity is defined as the capacity to interpret and act on one's own and others' feelings. These concepts are combined with the broad conceptualisation of health of the WHO, which includes multiple aspects. Health is a state of complete physical, mental, and social well-being, not merely the absence of disease (WHO, n.d.). This broad conceptualisation of health is combined with Wackerhausen's (1994) open concept of health, defined as the ability to meet goals and the quality of generalised capacity for action, stated as the relationship between the subject's goals, living conditions, and subject-action skills (Singla, 2015). Focusing on the broad context, including the living conditions, we discuss migration policies and the privileges or lack of them for the participants in our analysis. As part of the temporal context, COVID-19 and its consequences for the LATT couples are included in the analysis. Finally, we combine concepts such as digital emotions (Ellis & Tucker, 2011) with emotional reflexivity (Holmes, 2014) to explore how couples maintain emotional and sexual intimacy across distance, partly through online sexual activity, especially across national borders.

Our empirical study

The two cases highlighted in this chapter have been selected from a research project about the dynamics of transnationally distanced intimate relationships. They illustrate how the couples maintained intimacy, even in times of crisis, and reflect different sexual orientations embedded in diverse contexts and privileges. The original empirical study, conducted in 2017–2018, included semi-structured in-depth interviews (Kvale & Brinkmann, 2015) with 20 LATT couples. In view of the COVID-19 pandemic, we administered a follow-up survey in 2020–2021, to which 80% of our participants responded. The main inclusion criterion in the original and the follow-up study was partners constituting a couple living apart in different countries for at least one year due to work or education. Snowball techniques were used to recruit participants through the researchers' networks and relevant organisations. Email and phone were the primary means of giving participants study information and scheduling the interviews. The participants signed a consent statement and an agreement that the interviews would only be used for scientific purposes. We conducted most interviews in English but a few in Danish. Eight couples were interviewed online since the participants lived in different countries, while 12 were interviewed face-to-face in Denmark. Participant names are pseudonyms, based on the ethical rules for research of the Nordic psychological associations (Nordic Ethical Code, n.d.) to ensure anonymity and non-traceability. Compliance with GDPR regulations was ensured as the data were collected in the European Union.

The objective of the follow-up study was to explore the impact of COVID-19 on couples' relationships. We used the pandemic as a lens to understand LATT relationship dynamics under stress due to forced separation. We invited all 20 couples who participated in the original study to participate in a follow-up survey or a short online interview, and 70% of these took part. Two of follow-up interviews are presented in this chapter. Mette and David responded immediately and chose an online interview, while Theo sent a written reply. All the interviews were recorded and transcribed and have been presented elsewhere (Singla, 2024, in press), and subjected to a thematic analysis through close reading, meaning condensation, and interpretative strategies (Braun & Clarke, 2006). The interpretation goes beyond what is said directly in order to work out structures and relations of meaning not immediately apparent in the narrative. This interpretation requires a certain distance from what is said (Kvale, 1996). Six themes emerged from the analysis of the main and follow-up studies (Singla, 2024, in press), two of which are covered in this chapter. The first theme, from the main project, highlights *maintaining intimate relationships despite geographical distance,* and the second, from the follow-up study, focuses on the *impact of COVID-19 on couples' relationships, including their coping strategies.*

Selection of participants

The two cases differ in sexual orientation; the first couple was heterosexual, while the second was homosexual. The couples also differed in their geopolitical privileges, which involved immigration restrictions related to the couple's reunification. The first couple included a partner from the Global South (India), which is not strictly a geographical category, but more a replacement for development-oriented terms such as the 'developing world' or 'third world' and refers to an entire history of colonialism and neo-imperialism, also addressing spaces and peoples negatively impacted by globalisation (Clarke, 2022). In the second couple, both partners were from the Global North. However, both couples were from the upper middle class, having elements of choice and 'professional necessity' (Lindemann, 2019) as part of the reason for being a LATT couple.

The first case chosen for this chapter is Mette and Das, a LATT couple who had a 2½-year-long relationship at the time of the first interview. Mette and Das met through the online dating platform Tinder in 2014 while he was working in Denmark after completing his MBA from a Danish University. Mette had responded to Das' post on Tinder, and their very first meeting was successful. Mette currently lives in Copenhagen, whereas Das had to return to Delhi because of immigration restrictions on their living together in Denmark. We only interviewed Mette initially and in the follow-up study, where she conveyed Das' opinions.

The second case concerns Theo, a Norwegian man, and his American partner, David, both working in academia, who had been in a same-sex relationship since 2012. Theo lived in Copenhagen, Denmark, where he had studied and worked at a university. Theo and David initially met in New York and dated intensely for a month before Theo returned to Denmark. They were in a long-distance relationship for 1½ years until David found a position at a Danish university, which enabled them to cohabit in Copenhagen for four years. Their careers in different parts of the Global North entailed their living apart, although they also had work opportunities to live together in the same country when possible. We interviewed them separately face-to-face.

Maintaining intimate relationships despite geographical distance and immigration policies

This theme deals with the two couples' sustaining their relationship despite large distances and a time difference. Mette and Das had almost 7000 km between them and a 3½–4½ hours' time difference, while Theo and David had a distance of 6000 km and a six-hour time difference (Table 7.1).

'More comfortable but you still get the loneliness' (Mette and Das)

Immigration restrictions in Denmark resulted in Das not having a permanent residence permit, which meant that Das and Mette had been in a LATT relationship for the past 2½ years. Their primary strategies for sustaining their relationship were using digital technology and visiting each other's city every three months, along with building relationships with each other's extended family. The extent to which individuals' social networks engage in the relationship is one of the key factors in supporting the individual in dealing with various stressors that might arise during a transnational long-distance relationship (including feelings of loneliness, isolation, longing, insecurity, and structural barriers). According to our analysis, Mette and Das engaged in some emotional reflexivity. Despite a long relationship, Mette still found online communication as the 'hard part of their relationship' as she expressed 'feelings of sadness, being alone, and having difficulty in remembering her experiences of the day to share with her partner'. Her

Table 7.1 Case studies: Mette and Das, Theo and David

Name/Age /Gender/ Citizenship*	*Job*	*Civil status/ length of relationship in years*	*Current couple status*/ location*	*LATT years apart*/Location*	*Reuniting pattern*
**At the time of the interview*			**2021*	**At the time of the initial interview 2017/18*	
Mette, early thirties, F, Danish	Auditor	Couple	LATT	2½ years since 2014	3–4 times a year
Das, early thirties, M, Indian	Engineer	Approx. 7	Copenhagen – New Delhi	Copenhagen – New Delhi	
David, early thirties, M, American	University faculty	Couple	LATT again	1½ years in 2011–2012	Visit each other every second month
Theo, late thirties, M, Norwegian	University faculty	Approx. 10	Brussels –Copenhagen (lived together 2012–2019)	New York –Copenhagen	

experience contrasts with the 'privileging of digital emotions' described by Ellis and Tucker (2011), by implying that digital emotions do not satisfy at the same level as face-to-face encounters.

> Now I feel more comfortable about it because we've done it for two years. So you don't feel the same loss in the same way … of course, you still get the loneliness and the missing part. You miss the person, and you hate having to recall everything that happened throughout the day because you must remember to tell the other person what has happened. …

When questioned about their visiting pattern, Mette explained that Das' tourist visa allowed him to visit Denmark for only two to three months. Then he returned to India, where she visited him for brief periods. In addition to the travelling challenges, the time difference (3.5–4.5 hours) made synchronous FaceTime exchange difficult and influenced the quality of the emotional exchange between them. 'If I have a long day at work, I don't call him because then he's gone to sleep by the time I come back.'

She also expressed some dissatisfaction with asynchronous communication through written texts, in which spontaneous interaction and spontaneous emotional exchange were missing. '… I think you don't say things as fast when you're texting … and you get the emotion, but you don't blurt out your emotion immediately.'

However, Mette emphasised that the high frequency of their visits made the missing sexual relationship acceptable and gave her a subjective feeling of his presence. There was no mention of online sexual activity or sexting, which highlights the absence of conflicts during the periods of separation. The *cycles of departure, separation, and return* (Stafford, 2005) every three months for Mette and Das helped to maintain their relationship as they looked forward to their reunion.

> Since we see each other so frequently, it's actually doable not to have a sexual relationship for that time. Then we have messages that are more romantic and not the sexual part … I always feel like he's there somehow … However, [when] he's not there, we tend not to fight as much or have arguments as much as when we're together.

Mette also explained that LATT gave her autonomy, which she greatly appreciated, as it balanced fusion and independence, as described by Carter et al. (2016). She wanted to maintain her independence along with the couple's intimacy at a distance.

> LATT is hard, I miss him, but it's also okay. I'm still quite an independent person So I have my own life. Some of my friends throw themselves so much into being a couple that they forget themselves in it. I do have my own life and do my own things.

Moreover, the nationwide 'digital divide' also affected their interaction, as sometimes there could be a poor internet connection, perhaps due to electricity failure in India, which interrupted communication. 'I'm sitting there in the middle of telling a story, but then I can never finish the story because... .'

In summary, Mette's narrative shows that she could sustain an intimate relationship with Das, where they maintained their mental health and well-being, despite a large geographical distance, due to frequent online contact and being physically together every three months. However, she was also aware of the limitations of online interpersonal interaction, such as the lack of spontaneity and bodily intimacy, and the risk of interruption due to power failure.

'I need you here for me when you aren't here for me' (Theo and David)

Theo and David had planned for communication, managing different expectations, and sexual encounters with others, in order to maintain their intimate relationship and meet their needs in their relationship.

One arrangement was synchronous communication which made it possible to connect with each other's feelings and need for contact, while another was by eating together online. David narrated:

> I started to use Skype for him. (...) We would sometimes make a date. We would plan it because a six-hour time difference also makes a big deal... ., I get home around 7 pm my time, 1 pm your time (...) and maybe I'd have my dinner, and he'd have his lunch.

Digital media played a significant role in promoting 'digital emotions' by enhancing emotional bonding through online exchanges. The couple planned online dates to overcome the cycle of separation and to create a shared everyday activity.

From the start of their relationship, scheduling of contact had been important for Theo, who wanted them to agree on rules for regular contact. Theo elaborated his perspective on why clarity about rules for contact is crucial:

> You're not together every day, you don't have a concrete feeling of what the other person's doing, and there can be many instances of jealousy ... For me, it's more important to set some ground rules, where he wasn't going to be angry with me for not answering the phone immediately or for going out with friends and partying when he wasn't here.

The rule-setting prevented conflicts, jealousy, and misunderstandings, which affected their mental health and matched their expectations. Theo's quote shows that a lack of rules for contact can give rise to conflicting emotions if one cannot get in touch, illustrating emotional reflexivity and taking account of one's partner's feelings. LATT couples, like their cohabiting counterparts, might experience differences in their partners' need for contact and expectations. Digital media enabled Theo and David to overcome asynchronous contact, along with regular Sunday emails called 'Sunday Inzights'. These were emails that David would wake up to, full of different things that Theo wanted to share with him.

Compared to Theo's concerns about how their different personality factors played a role in navigating each other's feelings, David did not emphasise personality factors or jealousy. To illustrate interpersonal difficulties, David mentioned Theo's disappointment that David could not be available online the day Theo handed in his dissertation:

> He wanted to call me up and say that we'd see each other face-to-face and say yay! He wanted to read the acknowledgments because he thanked me for them.

For Theo, particular occasions needed to be prioritised with *face-to-face interaction*, while David emphasised being present where he was geographically and felt that *just greeting by text* was sufficient. This disagreement highlights the need to negotiate expectations for communication and ways to connect emotionally when partners are apart.

Another agreement of being in a LATT relationship for Theo and David involved having an open relationship. They did not have online sex when they were apart, instead having their needs for physical intimacy met by sexual encounters with others. According to McRae and Cobb (2020), long-distance couples are (more) open to discussing sexual and emotional boundaries in their relationship to benefit their relational and sexual health while being apart. This was also the case for Theo and David, and their discussions about the subject included feelings like (dis)trust, insecurity, and what it meant to be in an open relationship.

Theo and David's open relationship shows how LATT couples reshape the norms of an intimate relationship in creative ways so that open sexuality does not challenge the loyalty between LATT partners. Having an open relationship requires considerable navigation between boundaries and feelings. From the beginning, David and Theo agreed *not to be sexually exclusive* while maintaining emotional exclusivity by agreeing that they would not date another man more than once. To protect their relationship and avoid jealousy, they did not tell or ask the other about their sexual dating patterns.

An open relationship that polarises between physical and emotional intimacy requires a high level of emotional reflexivity from both partners, which reveals how an open relationship is much more than just a physical arrangement. Blasband and Peplau (1985) suggest that gay male relationships typically go through predictable stages in which an initial 'honeymoon' of sexual exclusivity is followed by a change to openness. The open sexual aspect provides them with bodily autonomy. For monogamous couples, sexual encounters with others could lead to distrust. However, for Theo and David, the open relationship created a balance in their LATT relationship while also meeting individual bodily needs.

In summary, David and Theo's story shows how they maintained an intimate relationship when apart transnationally by bonding emotionally with synchronous communication; this was an essential factor in how they manifested themselves as a couple while meeting individual needs. Despite their intention to set ground rules for how to communicate when living apart, they had to arrange communication on an ongoing basis, depending on the given situation. Most important was their reflexive negotiation of rules regarding sexual encounters with others, which required them to be emotionally exclusive to show loyalty to the other partner's feelings. The following theme highlights how the LATT couples coped with the global pandemic situation in the year 2020, which affected face-to-face meetings.

The impact of COVID-19 dynamics on the LATT couples' relationship and their coping strategies

The analysis highlighted the dominant aspects of this theme, leading to two subthemes: (1) uncertainty and (2) finding ways to cope with their challenges as a couple during COVID-19.

The uncertainty: Inability to plan

Mette's response to a question about COVID-19 emphasised the travel restrictions imposed globally by national regimes and her difficulty in scheduling the face-to-face meetings that she and Das had previously arranged for every second month. She explained:

> Yes, it's hard that we cannot plan when to see each other. Normally when we left each other, we always had the prospect of when we'd see each other again. It was about two months between each meeting … That hasn't been possible.

Against the backdrop of involuntary physical separation for almost eight months, Mette recollected the pleasant memories of their last face-to-face visit in Dubai with excitement and joy. She pinpointed her frustration about their inability to plan visits as strict lockdown and travel restrictions were imposed in both countries with no clarity about when they would end. The uncertainty is analysed as the major challenge. 'The problem is that we don't know when we'll see each other again … . We cannot plan. We can't just live through online communication.'

Mette is highly aware of the long-term stability of her LATT relationship with Das (5½ years at the time of the follow-up interview) and the feelings of sadness and missing Das are emphasised poignantly in Mette's narrative.

> ... we have done long-distance relations for a while, so it's easy for us. But we always had the prospect of seeing each other, which we don't have now. It's very hard ... . It comes in waves. Like you're living your life, doing your things. Then suddenly you realise he's not here. ... we use WhatsApp.

Mette also mentioned that she visited her family who live 70 km away in Denmark, whereas Das lived with his parents in Delhi, which helped him during the prolonged periods of isolation. When asked provocatively by the first author if she did not think about finding a boy next door, instead of having a partner 6000 km away, her explicit reply reflects her commitment to their relationship. Her optimism regarding the end of the pandemic is interpreted as one of the major strengths in her coping process. 'No, because that would be still more heart-breaking. All pandemics end, they don't last forever.'

On the other hand, for David and Theo, the contact situation during COVID-19 was radically different. Before the closing of the borders, David managed to get to Theo's place and stayed with him during the lockdown in Denmark in 2020. This was ideal for them because they were both able to work from home:

> We were extremely fortunate to have the resources and ability to make that happen. During the lockdown, we both worked from home (including online teaching), with surprising ease. In the past, we haven't been too good at both working from home at the same time.

During the COVID-19 situation, these two couples re-organised their ways of living and working together. This adjustment parallels research where couples have explored new ways of getting to know each other during COVID-19 in the Global North and the Global South, as demonstrated by Abrahamson (2021) and Ahuja and Khurana (2021).

The quote above also shows inequalities between LATT couples. In contrast to Mette and Das, the migration regime did not affect Theo and David when they wanted to visit each other. They are both from the Global North, living in European countries and privileged, unlike Mette and Das. However, they too expressed sadness at their inability to plan family visits due to border closures since March 2020, which affected their mental well-being and led to concerns about health-related safety.

> (...) a bit of imbalance in terms of who visits whom. A bigger challenge visiting our families – particularly in the US, but to some extent in Norway as well. We saw my family this summer but haven't seen his since December 2019 and might not see them until 2021.

We can sum up by concluding that unlike our first long-distance couple, Mette and Das, Theo and David managed to live together during lockdowns in 2020 due to their privileged work situation and their place in the Global North. COVID-19 compelled LATT couples to reconsider their visiting and living arrangements in times of uncertainty. For Theo and David, it was an opportunity to revisit what these arrangements meant for them as a couple and how to manage to live and work together, which worked out well, despite their previous experiences.

Finding ways out: Coping strategies

When questioned directly about how she was facing the COVID-19 situation, Mette fantasised about a setting without COVID-19 and described sharing books as their way to cope with the demands of involuntary separation over a prolonged period. Das was an avid reader, and recommended books for Mette to read, which became the subject of mutual discussion for them.

> Of course, we would have continued travelling back and forth, and had lots of adventures together. ... now it's mostly about which book to read ... it's Das who does most of the reading ... . Whenever he reads a book he thinks I would like, he recommends it to me. Then I read it, and we discuss it afterwards. 'Born a Crime: Stories from a South African Childhood', an autobiographical comedy book by the South African Trevor Noah is an example.

Mette further emphasised the significance of discussing a book during the days with limited everyday activities due to the lockdown. She also mentioned their experience of sharing music and mental health-promoting activities such as yoga, workouts, and recipes.

> At least you can talk about the book, what is happening in the book, and not much is happening in our lives these days. ... We still share music. One day we were sharing music with each other ... I tried to get Das to do some yoga; it would be good for him. But he's doing workouts for his squash from one of the best players on YouTube.

Lastly, she lamented the barrier to joyful shared activities, such as cooking a meal together, caused by the different time zones, thus pointing out a structural barrier to the optimal adaptation cycles of *departure, separation, and return* (Stafford, 2005). The COVID-19 travel restrictions further exacerbated these structural constraints and postponed Mette and Das' reunion for an unknown period. 'We like to cook together but we can't cook because of the time difference ... almost four hours. It would be weird for one of us, we just share recipes now.'

Mette summed up her suggestions for sustaining LATT relationships, even during COVID-19, through her reply to a question about advice to other

LATT couples based on her experiences, which involved emotional reflexivity and the online communication of emotions through shared meaningful activities to sustain mental health and well-being. 'I think it's important to have something you can talk about online ... maybe cooking, books or music. You do not have a normal life together ... You create your own little world in a different way.'

> Denmark has highly restrictive immigration policies for Indians. However, Mette and Das continued their LATT relationship through digital technology, sharing not only their everyday lives but also creative activities such as music, books, and yoga. We conclude that Mette was directly affected in her LATT relationship as COVID-19 led to international travel restrictions, preventing her face-to-face visits to Das in India.

At the beginning of COVID-19, David and Theo were apart, and the distance affected David emotionally just as when they had lived apart in the pre-COVID situation. During their forced separation, digital devices and social media provided a vital coping mechanism for handling loneliness and maintaining emotional rituals such as saying goodnight.

> Although I do feel lonely at times, cell phones and social media help me feel connected to my partner. I know that if I want to show him my new haircut, and wish him goodnight, he will be there with a response.

On the other hand, Theo acknowledged that being with his friends and having his own interests was always his lifestyle when he and David were apart. In that sense, COVID-19 did not change this LATT couple's individual activities that helped to fill up the time when they were away from each other.

Theo and David's situation improved once they were able to live together before the borders were closed, but their individual and social needs were constrained and made them find new ways of being sociable. As the statement below suggests, each partner's individual autonomy in normal daily life when living apart was also vital for them when they lived together as a couple:

> ... social life and travel are fundamental parts of who we are as individuals and as a couple. COVID-19 has definitively affected both. We miss going out in less restricted circumstances, and we miss travelling to new places and meeting new people. However, we try to manage that feeling of loss by seeing a small group of friends regularly and by exploring Copenhagen. In addition, we work [write] more than we did before.

The lockdown limited their opportunities for coping with the distance and thus affected the mental health of this LATT couple. Conversely, the COVID-19 situation gave Theo and David new possibilities for living and working together. This applied not only to the material aspects of their lives but also to the way they took care of their well-being as a couple and as individuals. During the COVID-19 lockdowns, limited social activities gave them flexibility in cultivating their individual interests. For them, the challenges were about safety and being unable to visit their family on another continent.

Discussion and conclusion

This chapter has presented how two LATT couples-maintained intimacy in their relationship before and during COVID-19, illustrating concrete ways in which LATT couples survived and how the lockdowns helped them to gain new insights into their intimate life. Existing knowledge related to COVID-19 is primarily at the macro level, such as the 6.7 million deaths (WHO, 2023), and the novelty of our chapter's contribution is the micro-level, process-oriented focus. The two cases provide a micro-level lens for COVID-19, showing how couples were compelled to find new ways of being in a relationship. Compared to couples living together who were suddenly forced to separate due to COVID-19, LATT couples did not suffer in the same way since they were already used to being apart and flexible and creative in maintaining their relationship. In that light, LATT couples showed how the lockdowns provided new insights into their intimate life.

The interactional states of being together and apart were intertwined, leading to mutual enabling and constraining of each other in multiple ways. Despite geographical distance, frequent online contact, planning to be together and having quality time together emerged as resources for maintaining an intimate relationship in the pre-pandemic times. During COVID-19, temporal and affective mobility were a burden, as demonstrated by Holmes (2014) and Carter et al. (2016). However, with its unique focus on LATT, this study pinpoints immigration legislation as a significant burden on couples, especially when one partner is from the Global North and the other is from the Global South.

Spouses may occupy various positions in social hierarchies depending on their nationality. Privileges and disadvantages are seen both in society and in the couple's relationship and are especially visible in the restrictive immigration policy for Das, as shown in the first case study. Many couples are forced into LATT status because of restrictive, draconian immigration policies and quotas that delay family reunification. One spouse may be working in the United States or Europe on a temporary work permit, while the other spouse is waiting for a visa in the country of origin – sometimes for years! In the United States, some LATT couples are not a 'voluntary' group, while others are dual-job couples with the privilege of choice, as highlighted by Lindeman (2019).

Optimal adaptation to the *cycles of departure, separation, and return* (Stafford, 2005) is vital to understanding how couples grow accustomed to a love life during their LATT period.

As the analysis shows, in the absence of a similar background due to their different nationalities, partners in LATT relationships create their own procedures through *reflexive negotiations* during separations, focusing on their common interests, such as sharing music, online dates, and asynchronous written texts such as the above-mentioned 'Sunday Inzights' weekly text written by Theo for David. Sharing their interests and thoughts through constructive activities promoted digital emotional connection while they were apart.

In line with the topic of the book, health is both a collective and individual concern that is vital for the sustainability of a society, and the findings in this chapter highlight mental health. Both couples created narratives about dealing with distance by using strategies such as mutual exchange to cope with the emotional disturbances that could affect their mental health and well-being. This involved discussing how to handle difficult feelings like distress and jealousy, which motivated these LATT couples to be emotionally reflexive since they could not see each other or know what the other person was doing. Another concrete example is the need to negotiate expectations for communication and ways to connect emotionally through digital technology when the partners were apart. Additionally, the same-gender couple also challenged the norms of how to maintain their relationship by agreeing to open sexual relations, thus not being sexually exclusive, while Mette and Das continued to be sexually exclusive. However, while the distance and time difference could challenge the couples, they also enabled them to maintain their individual autonomy, as concluded by Carter et al. (2016). On the other hand, their narratives about personal autonomy could have been describing a coping strategy to manage the time apart by reframing it in a positive light.

During COVID-19, as our research reveals, long-standing, stable LATT relationships activated different dynamics to counter time zone differences, immigration constraints and travel uncertainties that were affecting their mental health and well-being. Our findings also show how these couples survived in creative ways and lived with unexpected dynamics in their lives. The couples' ability to cope with the situation depended on their privileges and contextual possibilities, as demonstrated by David and Theo in the second case study. Even though COVID-19 was challenging, it also highlighted constructive aspects of how these LATT couples maintained their relationship.

We emphasise that the lives and relationship phases of LATT couples should be studied longitudinally to better understand the dynamics involved, especially conflicts affecting their mental health. The findings confirm that contextual and social factors, including the immigration laws of the host country, are key to strategies for coping and couple formation across borders (Singla & de Ponte, 2021; Singla & Runciman, 2019).

Implications for mental health policies and care providers

The number of LATT couples has increased exponentially in the 21st century, but the phenomenon is an understudied field in sociological and mental health literature. Numerous factors have caused the increase in LATT couples, the main ones being transnational migration triggered by changes in the labour market, global demand for highly qualified labour, and global income disparities prompting the search for better economic, educational, and career opportunities. Transnational migration is a strictly regulated policy in most countries, but in the United States and Denmark the joint migration of couples, married, cohabiting, or LATT, is restricted. Seldom are both partners given work permits or permanent residence status simultaneously, leading to the couple's separation in two different countries or continents. These separations are a cause of great stress for the individuals concerned. Yet little attention has been paid to the mental health burden that LATT couples must bear to sustain these relationships. Policymakers need to be aware of the toll on the mental well-being of partners who live in different countries. Enforced separations create a power differential among spouses that is often the underlying cause of domestic violence in immigrant families. Loneliness can aggravate substance abuse issues in one or both partners as a coping mechanism. A more compassionate approach to migration policies for LATT partners would benefit society as labour migration increases to the European Union and the United States.

LATT couples are here to stay as a new version of human relationships. Issues related to LATT lifestyles and stressors are not part of most mental health curricula. A lack of understanding and expertise regarding the LATT experience leaves mental health professionals ill-equipped to develop relevant services for LATT couples. Our study, partly conducted in the context of COVID-19, has shown that there is still much to learn about the resilience and adaptability of human relationships. Through an interdisciplinary, eclectic lens, our study underlines the necessity of critical scientific analysis in times of crisis and challenges, not only in Denmark but with a global outreach. The strategies described by our couples, Mette and Das, and David and Theo, highlight approaches that should be taught to mental health care workers providing psychosocial interventions, and in marriage and family counselling programmes. Our case studies show that the LATT couple relationship is a promising area for future research.

References

Abrahamson, A. (2021). More sex. Fewer fights. Has the pandemic actually been good for relationships? Retrieved September 2, 2021, from https://www.theguardian.com/us-news/2021/jul/11/couples-relationships-pandemic-romance

Ahuja, K. K., & Khurana, D. (2021). Locked down love: A study of intimate relationships before and after the COVID lockdown. *Family Relations*, *70*(5), 1343–1357.

Beck, U. U., & Beck-Gernsheim, E. (2013). *Distant love.* Polity Press.

Blasband, D., & Peplau, L. (1985). Sexual exclusivity versus openness in gay couples. *Archives of Sexual Behavior*, *14*(5), 395–412. 10.1007/BF01542001

Braun, V., & Clarke, V. (2006). Using thematic analysis in psychology. *Qualitative Research in Psychology*, *3*(2), 77–106.

Carter, J., Duncan, S., Stoilova, M., & Phillips, M. (2016). Sex, love and security: Accounts of distance and commitment in living apart together relationships. *Sociology*, *50*(3), 576–593.

Clarke, M. (2022). *Global South*. Retrieved August 30, 2022, from https://onlineacademiccommunity.uvic.ca/globalsouthpolitics/2018/08/08/global-south-what-does-it-mean-and-why-use-the-term/

Ellis, D., & Tucker, I. (2011). *Social psychology of emotion*. SAGE Publications.

Gerstel, N., & Gross, H. (1984). *Commuter marriage: A study of work and family*. Guilford Press.

Grover, S., & Schliewe, S. (2020). *Trailing spouses (India)*. Retrieved October 16, 2021, from https://www.in-formality.com/wiki/index.php?title=Trailing_spouses_(India)

Holmes, M. (2014). *Distance relationships: Intimacy and emotions amongst academics and their partners in dual–locations*. Palgrave Macmillan.

Holmes, M. (2019). 'Going against the grain'? Distance relationships, emotional reflexivity and gender. *Emotion, Space and Society*, *31*, 56–62.

Kobayashi, K., Funk, L., & Khan, M. (2017). Constructing a sense of commitment in 'living apart together' (LAT) relationships: Interpretive agency and individualization. *Current Sociology*, *65*(7), 991–1009.

Køppe, S. (2012). A moderate eclecticism: Ontological and epistemological issues. *Integrative Psychological & Behavioral Science*, *46*(1), 1–19. 10.1007/s12124-011-9175-6.

Kvale, S. (1996). *InterViews: An introduction to qualitative research interviewing*. SAGE Publications.

Kvale, S., & Brinkmann, S. (2015). *Interviews – Learning the craft of qualitative research interviewing*. SAGE Publications.

Li, Y., & Samp, J. A. (2021). The impact of the COVID-19 pandemic on same-sex couples' conflict avoidance, relational quality, and mental health. *Journal of Social and Personal Relationships*, *38*(6), 1819–1843. 10.1177/02654075211006199

Lindemann, D. (2019). *Commuter spouses: New families in a changing world*. Cornell University Press.

McRae, L., & Cobb, R. (2020). A qualitative analysis of themes in long-distance couples' relationship boundary discussions. *The Canadian Journal of Human Sexuality*, *29*(2), 212–220. https://www.utpjournals.press/loi/cjhs

Nordic Ethical Code for Psychologists. (n.d.). https://www.google.com/search?q=nordic+psychology+ethics&rlz=1C1GCEB_enDK995DK995&o

Parrenas, R. (2005). *Children of global migration: Transnational families and gendered woes*. Stanford University Press.

Rajkumar, R. P. (2020). COVID-19 and mental health: A review of the existing literature. *Asian Journal of Psychiatry*, *52*, 102066.

Reutschke, D. (2010). Living apart together over long distances – Time-space patterns and consequences of a late-modern living arrangement. *Erdkunde*, *64*(3), 215–226.

Singla, R. (2015). *Intermarriage and mixed parenting: Promoting mental health & wellbeing*. Palgrave Macmillan.

Singla, R. (2024, in press). *Living apart together transnationally (LATT) couples: Promoting mental health and intimacy.* Springer (under review).

Singla, R., & de Ponte, U. (2021). Love in the context of transnational academic exchanges: Promoting mental health and wellbeing. In C.-H. Mayer & E. Vanderheiden (Eds.), *International handbook of love: Transcultural and transdisciplinary perspectives* (pp. 599–620). Springer.

Singla, R., & Runciman, C. N. (2019). Den hvide side af det (etnisk) blandede Danmark: forhandlinger af køn, race og etnicitet i blandede parforhold [The White side of (ethnically) mixed Denmark: Negotiating gender, race and ethnicity in mixed couples]. In L. L. Hansen (Ed.), *Køn, magt & mangfoldighed* [Gender, power & diversity] (pp. 289– 314). Frydenlund.

Singla, R., & Varma, A. (2019). *LATT (Living apart together transnational) couples: Promoting mental health and wellbeing.* ICCP Keynote Conference, Bengaluru, India.

Stafford, L. (2005). *Maintaining long-distance and cross-residential relationships.* Routledge.

Valsiner, J. (2014). *An invitation to cultural psychology.* SAGE Publications.

Wackerhausen, S. (1994). Et åbent sundhedsbegreb – mellem fundamentalisme og relativisme [An open concept of health – Between fundamentalism and relativism]. In U. Juul Jensen & P. F. Andersen (Eds.), *Sundhedsbegreber* [Concepts of health]. Philosophia.

WHO (n.d.). *Health and well-being.* https://www.who.int/data/gho/data/majorthemes/health-and-well-being

WHO. (2023). *Pandemic deaths, 2023.* Retrieved January 17, 2023, from https://covid19.who.int/

Part 3

Urgent changes and sustainable solutions

Crisis as a gamechanger for sustainable development?

8 COVID-19

A disruption of interprofessional collaboration in health care

Sine Lehn

Introduction

Even before the first patient with COVID-19 was detected in Denmark, the COVID-19 health care regime was being developed, as hospitals were preparing to receive infected patients. The knowledge gained from the pandemic in southern Europe (Mapelli, 2020) meant that Danish hospitals were preparing for large numbers of critically ill patients, who needed to be isolated and treated (Hørlyk, 2021). Initially, it took several days to determine whether a patient was infected. Consequently, many patients had to be treated as if they were infected to avoid potential transmission of infection. Under emergency departments, assessment clinics, including video assessment clinics, were set up on the outskirts of hospitals to enable patients to have their temperature, pulse, and blood pressure taken without coming into close contact with other patients or health professionals. COVID hotlines, as well as contact tracing and monitoring units, were established, redeploying many health care professionals in addition to employing personnel with other types of qualifications.

More isolation and intensive care units were established along with special reception conditions for potentially infected persons. Despite this, the situation was characterised by great uncertainty and media fear that Denmark could face the same situation as northern Italy, where the bodies of COVID-19 patients were transported in military convoys. Health professionals were relocated to new functions, and some were transferred to acute care clinics from their usual positions in, e.g., outpatient care (many outpatient clinics were closed as part of the national lockdowns) or elective surgery.

An ambition of more and better collaboration across health care has been formulated by the WHO (WHO, 2010), which points to the global recruitment and retainment crisis as another focal argument for the strengthening of collaboration in health. The WHO also argues for a strategy of co-creation that invites civic society and others to enable the development of high-quality service delivery in health care.

This chapter explores how interprofessional collaboration (IC) changed during the COVID-19 health care regime. The following research questions guide the analysis:

DOI: 10.4324/9781003441915-11

> How did health professionals employed in the COVID-19 regime experience the IC in which they were involved? What governing logic can be identified based on the professionals' accounts? How were professional jurisdictions and power relations altered? The COVID-19 regime is particularly interesting in relation to the study of IC, because of its special status as both 'a part of' and 'different from' the ordinary health care system. The regime was set up and governed by health system structures and policies, but at the same time it formed a separate organization, entailing new practices that changed rapidly over the course of the pandemic. The circumstances surrounding the COVID-19 virus (e.g. the scarcity of protective equipment, the global insecurity and the initial lack of knowledge of the virus) in some ways sidelined the organizational and professional rules that usually form and govern IC in health care. This makes the study of IC as experienced by health professionals interesting because it provides insight into what happens to IC when, for a while, it is no longer possible to conduct 'business as usual'.

Due to the inaccessibility of the empirical field during the pandemic, research into the influence of COVID-19 on collaborative practices has been somewhat delayed. Currently, however, the body of knowledge is rapidly growing. Examples of studies that have inspired this chapter are Corruble and Paris (2020), who explore how care was transformed into telecare, and Bernild et al. (2021), who show the need for enhanced communication with relatives of COVID patients in intensive care. The chapter is also inspired by Khalili and Price (2021), who attempt to analyse and discuss the broader effects of the pandemic on IC based on sociological theory. The IC research community has on several occasions pointed out different aspects that would be particularly interesting to explore in future research (Goldman & Xyrichis, 2020; Khalili & Xyrichis, 2020). This chapter helps to answer questions raised by Goldman and Xyrichis in a special issue of the *Journal of Interprofessional Care*: How did COVID-19 lead to renegotiations of professional boundaries? What was the impact of COVID-19 on the system of professions, including professional hierarchies and power balances? (Goldman & Xyrichis, 2020).

Theory

The empirical analysis presented in this chapter is broadly informed by the sociology of professions and insights into the relationship between professions and power. Two scholars from this tradition have served as inspiration for the analysis of how power permeates IC, namely the sociologists Elliot Friedson (1923–2005) and Andrew Abbott (1948–). Friedson conceptualised how the professions in general terms can be said to represent a special kind of logic of governance, the logic of professionalism (Freidson, 1990, 2001). This logic is seen in conjunction with two other governing logics, the logic of the market and the logic of bureaucracy. Together they constitute an ideal regulative order of any given labour market, such as health care. Whereas the logic of the market has profit, competition, supply, and demand as its focal point, the logic of bureaucracy has quality assurance, documentation, and standardisation as its main interest. The logic of professionalism (in the case of clinicians) is based on professional knowledge and knowledge of the individual patient. Friedson, using the American health care system as his basis, argued that all three logics should be used in the development of the health care system. Each logic holds its own challenges, which is why they need to keep each other in check and thereby ensure a balance in considerations of economy/resources, patient needs, and sound administration of the whole system. Because the logics in many respects are in conflict, they will produce very different directions for development (Freidson, 1990, p. 439). Therefore, it must be decided which of the logics forms the primary basis for system development.

Secondly, the analysis is inspired by sociologist Andrew Abbott, who in his book *The System of Professions* (Abbott, 1988) elaborated on the idea that professions are joined together in an eco-system. Each profession in the system deals with different aspects of 'human problems' in need of professional assistance. Besides the idea that professions co-exist in an interdependent system, Abbott's major contribution to the sociology of professions is his exploration and conceptualisation of the ways in which different professional groups strive to demarcate their area of jurisdiction and achieve social closure. Abbott's work thus emphasises that professions are not neutral providers of 'services', but closely connected to hierarchies and negotiations of power on the macro, meso, and micro levels. This chapter focuses on exploring the meso- and micro-level negotiations as they are experienced by the professionals themselves. Here, the concept of positioning (Davies & Harré, 1990) is used to show how professions are positioned as central or peripheral in IC and how the COVID-19 regime made renegotiations of positions possible.

The notion of interprofessional collaboration

Interprofessional collaboration is a complex and multi-faceted practice. The literature offers a multitude of definitions. Previous research shows how health professionals attribute their own meaning to the term depending on their educational background and their individual work experience (Lehn, 2023). Following these insights, this chapter does not operate with a fixed conceptualisation of IC. Instead, the analysis explores the practices that the involved professionals themselves define as IC in order to provide an understanding of what constituted everyday collaborative practices in health care during COVID-19.

Method

The analysis in this chapter is based on six qualitative interviews with health professionals who were all employed in the COVID-19 health care regime (see Table 8.1 for an overview of the informants). They were recruited through a post on LinkedIn, and interviewed online by the author, who was unfamiliar with all of them. Four informants were employed in treatment units, one worked in a hotline unit and one in a contact tracing and monitoring unit. All those who replied to the post on LinkedIn were interviewed. This recruitment strategy made it possible to reach out to many potential informants who had a desire to talk about their experiences during COVID-19. One might expect professionals with extraordinary experiences, or those with strong opinions on the COVID-19 regime or IC, to come forward. The strategy also made it impossible to ensure equal distribution between different kinds of professionals. Consequently, no doctors participated, which is judged to be a weakness in this study.

All informants were informed about the aim of the research and gave their consent in writing. Interviews were conducted based on a semi-structured interview guide that focused on inviting informants to provide close descriptions of interprofessional collaborative practices throughout the first two years of the pandemic (2020–2022). Informants were also asked to reflect on their experiences. Interviews lasted from 30 to 60 minutes and were transcribed verbatim by a student employee. All names and places have been anonymised.

The analysis was conducted in a generally abductive manner (Alvesson & Kärreman, 2011). The first part of the analysis was conducted as part of the interviewing, as the informants were asked if the COVID-19 regime had provided them with new interprofessional collaborative experiences. All informants

Table 8.1 Informants included in the study

Name	*Profession*	*Position, pre-COVID*	*Position, during COVID*
Emma	Occupational therapist		Contact tracing and monitoring unit managed by the police
Peter	Nurse	Emergency unit, hospital	Emergency unit, hospital
Fatema	Physiotherapist	Infectious diseases unit	Infectious diseases unit turned into an intensive COVID unit, hospital
Celia	Nurse		Intensive COVID unit, new established
Vivian	Nurse	Gynaecologist unit	A semi-intensive COVID unit, hospital
Eva	Physiotherapist	Administrative unit, hospital	COVID hotline, hospital virus tester, test centre, hospital

confirmed this assumption. Secondly, after transcription of the interviews, I explored the ways in which IC was experienced during the COVID-19 regime. This part of the analysis was especially inspired by Abbott (1988) and particular attention was paid to identifying new and familiar divisions of work as well as arguments for new ways of collaborating. Power relations and negotiations of professional power were integrated in the analysis through a focus on decision-making practices, collaborative conflicts, and the emergence of new professional hierarchies. The third analytical step was to explore whether and how the logics proposed by Freidson (1990), or any other logics, could be detected in the informants' narratives of IC during COVID-19. This stage of the analysis revealed that the identified logics changed over the course of the pandemic, based on some but not all interviews. In other words, I explored which logics were given primacy in the contexts represented in the interviews and whether changes could be identified.

Analysis

Collapse of the familiar

> For the first six months, everything was so new. It was chaos in the unit. To put it nicely. That is, the nurses didn't know what to do. We physiotherapists didn't know what to do either, apart from giving some pulmonary physiotherapy, of course. We also had to try out the new k-CPAP, the continuous CPAP. And we had to try it with a completely different virus than what we were used to. On top of that, patients were isolated …

This quote is from Fatema, a young physiotherapist. Prior to the pandemic, she specialised in pulmonary physiotherapy. This competency gave her an important role in the COVID-19 regime. Here, Fatema talks about how the unknown virus challenged the everyday familiarity of clinical practice, as well as her physiotherapy skills. The unit was faced with a group of patients who required a new form of oxygen therapy (continuous CPAP). Professionals recruited to positions related to hotlines and contact tracing also experienced a new form of working life, as most of them were not used to being employed in the same jobs as colleagues who were not health professionals. Emma, an occupational therapist with a master's degree, worked in a tracing and monitoring unit. She explained:

> I found it quite amazing that you can have health professionals, the police, and you can have all sorts of mixed operators. We had people who had studied Russian at university, we had people with autism, who were living at home, but could cope with talking on a phone for a few days a week. We had flight attendants and pilots employed as infection detectors. And team leaders, who weren't really leaders, but made sure the day-to-day operations ran smoothly by making sure that if there was some new

> knowledge that needed to get out to all the employees quickly, they were on the floor ready to take on that task. And I thought it was cool to see so many different backgrounds in one workplace. The fact that you can accommodate so many different people and bring so much diversity to the table …

The COVID-19 regime provided new tasks and new working conditions. Some informants worked with new colleagues, some of whom had non-health care qualifications. Their immediate experience was positive; much more could be done than they had imagined beforehand. They experienced uncertainty, but also excitement and energy.

New competencies and transformations of IC

One of the major challenges at the beginning of the epidemic in Denmark was the lack of protective equipment. In inpatient care, this meant rethinking which and how many professionals should enter the patient's room. Otherwise fixed divisions of labour between professions had to be revisited: for example, nurses started performing ECG tests based on rapid training by colleagues, thus taking over tasks traditionally assigned to others. Peter, a nurse working in the emergency unit, described this as a shift in the focus of IC:

'Suddenly, you discovered that you started from the patient and it's not the professional groups who have to go in and out 20 times with their own little thing.'

Peter found that the mantra of patient-centredness, often connected to IC (e.g. by D'Amour & Oandasan, 2005), suddenly became a reality. It was no longer the professional jurisdictions but the needs of the patient that guided the distribution of tasks. Fatema also recounted how she and her physiotherapist colleagues were given tasks that before COVID-19 were outside the jurisdiction of their profession:

> Suddenly, we weren't just physiotherapists. We were involved in many other treatments too because we were there in the patient's room. In the beginning, we had to economize on isolation gear. So, when I would go in and give k-CPAP, the nurse or the technicians … or the doctor, for example, could ask me to do some things, so they wouldn't have to go in and do it themselves, you see? So, we relieved each other a lot. And we got other skills in addition to what we knew (…) … one example was medicine. I could think of that, well, fortunately I have a background as a social and health care assistant too, but you could say my other colleagues who don't have that background, they were asked to empty the catheter bag, for example. And just, you know, like put it in a flask and hand it over to the nurse. So, all those things that we normally wouldn't do as physiotherapists, we did them.

Notably, it was the lack of protective equipment that enabled a patient-oriented collaborative practice; the professionals did what was needed when they were in the patient's room anyway. However, the experience of Fatema clearly illustrates that there was not a complete dissolution of professional jurisdictions. There were still boundaries and careful consideration about the distribution of tasks. When Fatema, as a physiotherapist, administered medication, it was because she was also a qualified social and health care assistant, which gave her a certain level of competence regarding medication. The urine sample was collected by the health care worker present in the patient room, but afterwards it was handed to the nurse for further action. Vivian, a nurse, explained how core competencies, including highly specialised ones, influenced the division of labour in her COVID unit, and suddenly a wide, unpredictable range of professional competencies was available:

> The great thing about being part of the first wave was that there was a huge willingness to try to solve the tasks together. We had the pulmonary nurses in our unit, who had experience with something similar to A-gas, which I wasn't familiar with. But people weren't shy about saying 'I don't actually know about this'. Neither were the doctors. That surprised me quite a lot, because I have often had to deal with doctors who said they were completely on top of what was going on, without actually knowing very much. But there were also new young doctors who were like 'I don't know what to do' and then some of the nurses would be like 'Well, I think we should do this and that', and then we would come up with some interim solutions. So I found people were really willing to try to work across the team constellations. It was amazing to be part of that.

These examples suggest the emergence of flexible, openly communicating IC that on the one hand is forced by circumstances to dissolve well-established professional boundaries, but on the other hand makes visible and draws on the competencies of the professionals in temporary teams. This indicates the existence of two governing logics: a professional and a pragmatic logic. IC was formed by the joint examination of the team's competencies, which developed during COVID-19:

> We've been inside each other's hearts during COVID. Now we know what our strengths are and what our weaknesses are, too. As physiotherapists, for example, we haven't really worked closely with death before. This experience of being with a patient and they suddenly go into cardiac arrest ... it happened often during COVID. We really learned a lot from the nurses and from the supervision sessions we had as well. (Fatema)

The circumstances surrounding the treatment of COVID-19 patients meant that the professionals had 'been inside each other's hearts'. The heart metaphor indicates that the professionals came very close to each other as human beings and as professionals. Fatema and her physiotherapist colleagues developed new skills in dealing with cardiac arrest and death, which they gained through intensified collaboration with nurses. The boundaries separating the professions and their work from each other were dissolved to a high degree and new competencies were learned from the repertoire of other professions. Learning between professions was reciprocal:

> (…) we also trained the nurses to give k-CPAP. If they were going in, or if we could see from that window that the nurse was in there, we would ask: 'Would you please, when you've finished with the patient, give him the k-CPAP mask? I'll watch from the outside'. So, we shared the work and trusted that they did …, that they could manage, you know. We trusted each other, even if you're not a physiotherapist for example, [or … even if] you're not a nurse, or you're not a doctor, etc. (Fatema)

There seemed to be a close link between the fact that everyone found themselves in new and unfamiliar situations and the rise of new forms of IC. A great deal of goodwill emerged in establishing new interprofessional collaborative practices that challenged the traditional boundaries between different professional groupings:

> In general, there was a real team spirit, because everyone was in a place where they weren't used to being. So the environment was new, so nobody necessarily knew where … where to find everything in the cupboards. There were coordinators who could help. But otherwise, people were from all specialities, and then there was a lot of interprofessional work. There were physiotherapists present all the time, helping to support the patient's breathing. And it was great that they were right there. (Celia)

Several informants agreed with research findings (Goldman, 2020) in reporting a very special atmosphere in the COVID regime.

New positions

In addition to the special atmosphere and sense of community of IC during the initial epidemic phase, the quote from Celia points to the changes in the positions of physiotherapists in the IC that emerged. The profession went from a peripheral to a central position in IC. Physiotherapists became more powerful in the sense that their professional competencies gained legitimacy and status. The change implied that the profession could engage in patient care in new ways and it provided an experience of mutual professional learning. Interviews from the emergency unit and the infectious disease unit confirm this shift:

> It has been an eye-opener, from COVID, what we could do and what you can do as a physiotherapist. I'm talking about our professional group. The

> fact that the other professions see the advantage of having physiotherapists on a regular basis [in the unit] ... 'Great that we can get help from the physiotherapists' ... Before COVID it was more like 'Well that's one professional group, they do their things'. (Fatema)

It is perhaps not surprising that physiotherapists most clearly gained a new position in the IC of the COVID-19 regime, as COVID-19 patients needed pulmonary physiotherapy. Yet this also reveals how IC in a hospital context often reflects a traditional clinical structure that positions nurses and doctors in the centre and other professions in the periphery.

Collaboration between colleagues?

As mentioned, the pandemic gave rise to many new tasks. Thousands of people were employed in contact tracing and monitoring units, hotlines, and vaccine units. Emma, an occupational therapist employed in a contact tracing and monitoring unit, narrated:

> There were retired doctors who thought it was interesting, who just came in and were part of the contact tracing and monitoring unit. And physiotherapists and ... so really many different health professional backgrounds were there as operators, also as health professional supervisors. And of course, in the beginning there was a certain hierarchy because you went to those who had a medical background if you felt unsure. But soon, some of us, who had some experience, were labelled supervisors, and then it was really more like: 'Well, are you a supervisor or are you an operator?' that formed the collaboration.

New job categories emerged. It was not necessarily a person's professional background that determined who had the competence to clarify professional uncertainty in the hotline unit. Initially, most staff were health professionals, but as the pandemic surged onwards and upwards, many non-health professionals were recruited, and some of these were also involved in aspects of care and treatment. Peter explained how the emergency department hired young people of secondary school age, giving them the tasks of greeting patients and holding their hands, and packing special kits with typical COVID-19 equipment.

After a few months 'on the floor' in the contact tracing and monitoring unit, Emma was promoted to supervisor and then to education officer. She thus quickly became part of the organisational development, and found that the monitoring and contact tracing unit changed from mainly hiring health professionals to taking people with all kinds of backgrounds and giving them ever shorter training courses:

> Some weeks 500 people were onboarded in one week. It went extremely fast. Normally they had 2–3 days of teaching and then two days of

> practical training afterwards. And when we onboarded the 500 that were scheduled to have three days of training, it was cut to two days, and it ended up being one day. They knew practically nothing when they started answering the calls. It was terrible. They weren't health professionals, so the whole thing of assessing or guiding people about a disease, when you don't have the basic understanding of it, it was really, really difficult for many of them as well. (Emma)

For Emma, it was frustrating to witness the change that led to a practice where non-health professionals were advising infected and potentially infected citizens on how to handle risks of illness and infection. She saw how the training courses were deteriorating, and it pained her because she felt that this compromised the quality of the advice offered. The point here is that the change entailed a transformation from a practice based on a combination of available professional knowledge, guidelines, and professional judgement to a hands-on practice based on guidelines and knowledge taught for the purpose. If the 'operator' or 'supervisor' had access to the knowledge base created and the latest guidelines, he/she was, from the perspective of the organisation, equipped to do the job. But not from Emma's perspective. The experience of interpreting a patient's symptoms, talking to people who are anxious, and the sense of the overall situation had been removed from the professional task. A picture of deprofessionalisation emerges. Eva, a physiotherapist, who was relocated to a test centre, shared how she felt about learning to perform the throat swab test with no prior experience:

> … in the beginning, our instructions were quite elaborate, something like, you know, we're going to go out here on one side, then on the other side and then down behind the bubble and so on. And then it ended up, (…) it was just like, you were just touching one side, and that was it. I thought, like with a lot of health care, well, it's something specialized, and you know the quality of this kind of procedure, I thought there must be some waste if you do it technically wrong, or you touch people's tongues or something, you know. I expected it to be a very complicated task, but it wasn't at all, as it turned out. (Eva)

Eva learns that testing is not very specialised or complicated after all. Her experience contrasts with that of Emma, who reported a decline in quality due to a simplification of the health care foundation of the work. This points to a new battlefield: Which competencies and tasks belong to the realm of health professionals, and which do not? What can be done (adequately) by anyone with a single day's training? The system of professions is threatened. Power negotiations are no longer limited to an interprofessional matter, it is now also an issue between colleagues.

Re-establishing the old system of professions

The second wave of the pandemic meant that some work practices in the COVID-19 regime returned to familiar divisions of labour and to the familiar professional hierarchies. The nurse Peter recalled how he found that the 'we're-all-in-the-same-boat' atmosphere in the emergency department was replaced by increasing irritation and 'petty fights' between the professions:

> Now that we were ... finding our way back to normal, there were some things we could hold on to, but there were also things where (...) e.g. the physiotherapist said, e.g. personal hygiene, they won't do that. So they had to discuss it with the nurses, that it was our job. They can accompany a patient to the toilet if they are doing training or mobilization anyway, but that's not ... but that's the limit.

As COVID-19 turned into an everyday matter, the boundaries between professions were re-established through continuous micro negotiations. Accompanying a patient to the toilet was traditionally a task for nurses, according to the physiotherapists, and they re-established the boundary there. The fact that this was the task the physiotherapists refused to keep doing can be seen as anything but coincidental. Health care involving bodily excretions have at all times been pushed away: first from doctors to nurses and later from nurses to social and health care workers (Lehn-Christiansen & Holen, 2019). Instead of helping each other or focusing on the patient's needs, IC returned to the familiar battle of core competencies. However, in the context of testing, contact tracing, and monitoring, the opposite tendency seemed to prevail; here, professional competencies and boundaries became less prominent during the course of the pandemic. There were no well-established boundaries and task distributions, i.e. no professional system, to return to.

Competing governing logics

Examining the development that took place in the contact tracing and monitoring unit from the perspective of Friedson's three logics makes it clear that all the logics were at play. The economic logic made efforts to keep costs down by hiring the cheapest personnel as the organisation grew, the professional logic tried to ensure adequate quality of services by installing health professionals as educators, while the bureaucratic logic attempted to provide contact tracing and monitoring units all over the country. However, the balance of power between the logics seemed to change during the pandemic. Emma described how she experienced this development in infection detection:

> As the epidemic developed, there was less focus on the medical side. It kind of fell into the background. We had a chief medical officer, and then

> we had one more doctor, who was kind of in charge of all the health professionals. And it was very frustrating for them that it didn't matter anymore, that we didn't stick to the health care part of it. But they didn't care that it was all a bit ... laissez faire and what the quality should be. The conditions under which people worked were also thrown around a bit, depending on how the epidemic developed. So in that way it's a whole different way of working, because you're used to a job going in certain rhythms, and then you might expand, but having to scale up and down so much, and focusing a lot on the fact that now it's a dangerous disease, and suddenly it's not so dangerous, and we're pretty safe and now we really only want employees with a clerical background, because they're cheaper and easier to get rid of. This shift was quite extreme. It's been difficult for many health professionals to cope with. Because you're sort of used to being at the top, aren't you? We were the base, and we expected that when we finished the epidemic, you would be left with the health professionals, because we were the ones at the core of it.

Emma described how she felt about her original position as 'the core' of the unit being taken over by clerical staff. This change can be seen as an expression of a shift in the balance of power between the governing logics. The logic of professionalism lost ground to both the logic of the market and to the logic of bureaucracy. The logic of professionalism was taken over by the logic of bureaucracy because the service provided to citizens was described and thus standardised to such an extent that the professional's discretion could be replaced by simple question and answer training and brief guidelines. Clerical staff were both cheaper and easier to get rid of than health professionals. This was smart when there was a need to up- and downscale the organisation on a regular basis. According to Emma, the shift from the logic of professionalism to the logic of the market had a profound impact on collaboration in the unit:

> We helped each other. At the same time, we were at war with each other to get the good jobs, the important tasks and so on, you see? So, it was such a ... weird job, where everything kept changing. You were always competitors, and it ended up being the health professionals versus the non-health professionals ...

Emma was involved in the establishment of one contact tracing and monitoring unit after another throughout the country. Without realising it, she and her health professional colleagues were making themselves redundant. In this way, her experiences were fundamentally different from those of professionals working in the COVID-19 regime in a hospital context. Instead of getting 'into each other's hearts' and mutually learning from each other, the differences between the health professionals and the non-health professionals were reinforced and the collaboration became a battleground marked by self-justification and fear of losing one's job. The logic of the market prevailed. This experience confirms Friedson's point that the primary logic affects several aspects of work, including collaboration, which is impaired when those who are supposed to work together are essentially turned into competitors.

Concluding remarks

This chapter has explored interprofessional collaboration (IC) as it took place in the COVID-19 regime of the Danish health care system during the first two years of the pandemic. It is argued that it was particularly interesting to explore IC as it played out in this regime, because of the special status of the regime as both 'part of' and 'different from' the ordinary health care system. An empirical analysis was based on six interviews with professionals and guided by these research questions:

How did health professionals employed in the COVID-19 regime experience the IC in which they were involved? What governing logic can be identified based on the professionals' accounts? How were professional jurisdictions and power relations altered?

The analysis, conducted with inspiration from Freidson (1990, 2001) and Abbott (1988), has shed light on how a new and flexible IC emerged in the initial phase of the pandemic. Patient treatment and care were provided with little or no consideration of hierarchies and established structures and were governed by two logics: a professional and a pragmatic logic. As a result, the professionals found that mutual learning and patient-centeredness were more prominent than in pre-pandemic health care. However, as the pandemic became part of everyday life, traditional professional boundaries and professional hierarchies seemed to be widely re-established. Despite this, the analysis suggests the finding that physiotherapists may have improved their position in IC on a more permanent basis. Further research is needed to firmly establish this as a fact.

The COVID-19 regime also included a hotline service, vaccine units, and contact tracing units. In this part of the regime a new collaborative landscape emerged, involving close collaboration between health professionals and employees with other qualifications. The analysis shows that the logics of professionalism, the market, and bureaucracy, as defined by Friedson, were at play, ensuring quality, cost-efficiency and country-wide services, respectively. However, as COVID-19 evolved, the logic of professionalism seemed to lose ground to the logic of the market and the logic of bureaucracy. Health professionals were to a large extent replaced with clerical workers and training activities were cut to a minimum. This shift was made possible due to short training courses and an increase in hands-on work.

In conclusion, the chapter demonstrates the need for further discussions of how and on what basis IC in health care should be developed. The experiences gained from the changes in collaborative practices during COVID-19 demonstrate the potentials for developing the more flexible and patient-centred IC that arises when health professionals are 'released' from the restrictions placed on them by 'ordinary' structures of the health care system. However, they also indicate a need for deep consideration of managerial and health policy aspects. The chapter shows that IC cannot run on professionals' enthusiasm and good-will alone. Careful thought about the nature of governing structures as well as about health care quality is clearly called for when new collaborative practices are developed. That applies to IC in both pandemic and post-pandemic times.

References

Abbott, A. (1988). *The system of professions: An essay on the division of expert labor*. University of Chicago Press.

Alvesson, M., & Kärreman, D. (2011). *Qualitative research and theory development. Mystery as method*. SAGE Publications Ltd.

Bernild, C., Missel, M., & Berg, S. (2021). COVID-19: Lessons learned about communication between family members and healthcare professionals—A qualitative study on how close family members of patients hospitalized in intensive care unit with COVID-19 experienced communication and collaboration with healthcare professionals. *Inquiry*, 4695802110600–469580211060005.

Corruble, E., & Paris, F. (2020). A viewpoint from Paris on the COVID-19 pandemic: A necessary turn to telepsychiatry. *Journal of Clinical Psychiatry*, *81*(3). 10.4088/JCP.20com13361

D'Amour, D., & Oandasan, I. (2005). Interprofessionality as the field of interprofessional practice and interprofessional education: An emerging concept. *Journal of Interprofessional Care*, *19*(Suppl 1), 8–20. 10.1080/135618205 00081604

Davies, B., & Harré, R. (1990). Positioning – The discursive production of selves. *Journal for the Theory of Social Behaviour*, *20*(1), 43–63.

Freidson, E. (1990). The centrality of professionalism to health care. *Jurimetrics*, *4*, 431–445.

Freidson, E. (2001). *Professionalism: The third logic*. Wiley.

Goldman, J., & Xyrichis, A. (2020). Interprofessional working during the COVID-19 pandemic: Sociological insights. *Journal of Interprofessional Care*, *34*(5), 580–583. 10.1080/13561820.2020.1806220

Hørlyk, U. (2021). *Akutlægens dagbog: hvad jeg lærte om mig selv, mens jeg forsøgte at redde andre* [The diary of an emergency doctor: What I learned about myself while trying to save others]. People's Press.

Khalili, H., & Price, S. L. (2021). *From uniprofessionality to interprofessionality: Dual vs dueling identities in healthcare*. 10.1080/13561820.2021.1928029

Khalili, H., & Xyrichis, A. (2020). A longitudinal survey on the impact of the COVID-19 pandemic on interprofessional education and collaborative practice: A study protocol. *Journal of Interprofessional Care*, *34*(5), 691–693. 10.1080/13561820.2020.1798901

Lehn, S. (2023). *Tværprofessionelt samarbejde i sundhedsfaglig praksis* [Interprofessional collaboration in healthcare practice] (2nd ed.). Munksgaard Danmark.

Lehn-Christiansen, S., & Holen, M. (2019). Ambiguous socialization into nursing: Discourses of intimate care. *Nurse Education Today*, *75*, 1–5. 10.1016/j.nedt.2019.01.002

Mapelli, M. (2020). What Covid is taking away from us: Cardiologist Dr Massimo Mapelli from Milan, Italy, discusses personal experiences from the 'front line' of this viral pandemic. *European Heart Journal*, *41*(22), 2053–2055. 10.1093/eurheartj/ehaa374

WHO (2010). *Framework for action on interprofessional education and collaborative practice*. World Health Organization. http://www.who.int/hrh/resources/framework_action/en/

9 Digital vigilance

Learnings from the COVID-19 pandemic

Christopher H. Gyldenkærne, Christine F. Bech, Aisha Malik, Troels Mønsted, and Jesper Simonsen

Introduction

When the COVID-19 pandemic struck during the winter and spring of 2020, the healthcare system needed an urgent transformation to bring about an effective response. This included establishing procedures and technological support to enable the diagnosis, treatment, and isolation of patients infected with the virus, safeguarding the public against infection during healthcare visits and protecting healthcare staff from exposure to infection. This in turn required the Danish healthcare sector to adopt rapid digital initiatives. COVID-19 initiated a digital change *force majeure* to ensure the rapid adoption of new digital solutions, adaptation of existing systems and development of new digital workflows.

Based on three case examples that unfolded during 2020–2021, the purpose of this chapter is to investigate how these rapid digital changes took place. It presents an analysis of the factors that facilitated and impeded the ability of actors within the healthcare system to be vigilant towards new emerging needs imposed by COVID-19 and to quickly develop and release digital support for new activities and workflows. This analysis highlights how human capabilities, the procedures for digital change, and the socio-technical context conditioned the digital crisis response.

Digital change in healthcare is known to be extremely complex and time consuming. Such change relates to the *information infrastructure*, defined as 'a shared, open, heterogeneous and evolving socio-technical system of Information Technology (IT) capabilities' (Hanseth & Lyytinen, 2010, p. 1). Information infrastructures in healthcare are typically constituted by large electronic health record (EHR) systems as well a significant number of other adjacent digital information systems that together enable the accumulation, distribution and usage of information and communication and the coordination of activities. This creates a complex *installed base* consisting of IT systems, practices, and conventions (Aanestad et al., 2017). Hanseth and Lyytinen (2010) defined an installed base as 'a set of IT capabilities and their user, operations and design communities' (p. 4).

DOI: 10.4324/9781003441915-12

In the healthcare context, the installed base for digital change consists of existing health information systems, users, their practices, such as dispensing practices, diagnostic procedures, etc., and the regulations that govern these. This pre-existing environment may provide opportunities, but it can also limit the freedom of digital change, since new infrastructure additions will inherently wrestle with the inertia of the installed base (Herbig & Kramer, 1993). Aanestad et al. (2017) stressed that 'studies of information infrastructures emphasize the durability and central role of existing practices, conventions, tools and systems, and this "installed base" is seen to fundamentally impact the evolution of information infrastructures' (p. 28). As a consequence, digital change involves extending the installed base through incremental change, for instance by adapting existing infrastructure components to serve new uses, and this process must involve close attention to how these new additions fit into or affect the installed base (Hanseth & Lyytinen, 2010).

In the Capital Region of Denmark (Region H) and Region Zealand (Region S), two of Denmark's five healthcare regions, EPIC,[1] a comprehensive EHR system, forms the backbone of the information infrastructure. Until COVID-19, the development of the information infrastructure was based on a plan-driven and release-based governance model whereby digital changes were carefully planned, developed, tested, and released in batches (i.e., rolled out and made available to all users across the two regions concurrently) every six months (Bansler, 2019, 2021). As this frequency shows, in healthcare, the development process for information infrastructure typically has a long-term orientation. In contrast to this, projects that develop or procure stand-alone applications are often managed with the intention of reaching closure (implementing a final version of the application) within a short timespan. In terms of digital change, one may observe a difference in infrastructure time (the long-term, open-ended, and incremental evolution of an infrastructure) and project time (projects deploying stand-alone applications seeking short-term closure) (Karasti et al., 2010).

Since the COVID-19 pandemic necessitated immediate digital changes to accommodate the new circumstances, it introduced a new and much shorter time-frame for the evolution of infrastructure. This disrupted the existing procedures for creating, releasing, and governing changes in the information infrastructure. Rapid digital changes were conducted by maintaining a top-down approach with swift region-wide roll-outs combined with high levels of standardisation across all clinical specialisms and their clinical practices. The focus shifted from the long-term incremental evolution of infrastructure to immediate closure in order to create and implement solutions that would enable the necessary crisis response.

Digital vigilance during COVID-19

The ability of organisations to overcome challenges imposed by their environment, often referred to as *resilience,* has long been of interest to researchers in the field of information systems and related sciences (Barasa et al., 2018; Vogus & Sutcliffe, 2007). While many partially overlapping definitions of this concept exist, resilience is generally understood as 'the ability [of a system] to sense, recognize, adapt, and absorb variations, changes, disturbances, disruptions, and surprises' (Bhamra et al., 2011, p. 5380). At an organisational level, resilience is typically presented as an emergent property of complex adaptive systems defined through a range of organisational variables, including 'material resources, preparedness and planning, information management, collateral pathways and redundancy, governance processes, leadership practices, organizational culture, human capital, social networks and collaboration' (Barasa et al., 2018). Recent research has indicated a correlation between the use of agile processes and the ability of organisations to achieve resilience (Baskerville & Pries-Heje, 2021).

The concept of resilience, along with the related body of theory, primarily highlights the organisational features and governance structures that bolster an organisation to manage quick transitions. COVID-19 initiated an unforeseen situation in the healthcare sector, which had no ready capability to withstand or quickly recover amid the new demand for swift digital transitions. In our study, *digital vigilance* emerges analytically as a collective term to describe this situation. We use digital vigilance as the empirical theme of this chapter to indicate the unexpected situation caused by COVID-19 and to explicitly focus on the perspective of the practitioners who drove the change and the conditions that enabled and constrained their ability to identify and quickly act upon the need for change. Digital vigilance points to the need for alertness and attentiveness and a complex collection of human capabilities, procedures for digital change and sociotechnical elements that enable practitioners to act to make urgent digital change take place successfully. Hence, we asked the following questions: (a) What human, technological, and organisational preconditions were present for the unforeseen rapid development and adoption of digital solutions across clinical specialisations? (b) What can we learn from this? (c) How can digital vigilance be maintained to meet future needs for urgent digital change?

In the following, we illustrate three real-world examples of digital vigilance. Based on these example cases and the insights, learning and implications that we draw from them, we then discuss how the conditions for digital vigilance can be improved in the event of future crises.

Three real-world examples of digital vigilance

The following three cases particularly attracted our interest because they exemplify the different implications and distinct characteristics of digital vigilance.

At the onset of the COVID-19 pandemic, the authors of this chapter had each been engaged in research projects in the healthcare sector that focused on digital change and innovation. However, because of COVID-19, these projects were temporarily paused. Nevertheless, the authors were able to closely witness and follow first-hand how COVID-19 disrupted ongoing routines for digital change. During this time, we maintained physical access to our regional office spaces, EHRs and other systems, internal communications, documents, newsletters, etc. This aroused our deep interest in how the regional and national health IT governance structures had been affected and how the demand for urgent change was being handled in clinical practices.

The cases emerged and had rapid uptake during COVID-19 as organisational initiatives encouraged by management as ways of handling the pandemic. Each case was observed and documented through informal talks and meetings and by interviewing key stakeholders (management, clinicians, developers, IT support) as well as through our access to internal regional systems and documentation. The three cases all addressed the need for swift transitions that aimed to support the main goals of providing care for patients in times of crisis, but they also differed from each other by having different criteria for development, implementation, roll-out, user adoption, ongoing improvements, etc.

Video consultancy: Adoption of digital solutions from the installed base

The emergence of the COVID-19 pandemic created an urgent need for swift transitions on many levels, including how typical doctors' appointments could be conducted both in hospitals and at general practitioners' surgeries. Shortly after the first wave of COVID-19, Danish public health experts and governing figures in healthcare pointed out the need to minimise as broadly as possible the exposure of healthcare staff both to each other and to patients. Scenarios of healthcare staff being infected across whole specialities or hospitals were considered likely, and thus alternatives to the established patient-doctor appointments system were explored and later implemented.

Before COVID-19, clinicians had been testing video consultancy technology in pilot projects at various clinics in Region H. That project had shown mixed results in terms of adoption. It presented itself as a controversial socio-technological change to the existing clinical practice of seeing patients in person for diagnosis, treatment, and follow-up care in full accordance with studies and literature evaluating digital consultancy technology (Kitamura & Wong, 2010; Stommel et al., 2019; Sturt et al., 2020). The region envisioned that the technology would improve healthcare expenditure and give patients more flexibility in their communication with healthcare staff. Since the region's organisational vision of digitalising more healthcare services had challenged the existing ways of providing care, especially for chronic patients, the use of video consultancy had generally remained low.

The digital video consultancy tool was one of the first digital initiatives in Region H to meet the need for distance solutions in daily healthcare operations. COVID-19 introduced the unprecedented need to keep doctors and patients apart to the greatest extent possible; all non-critical doctor's appointments were transitioned onto online meeting technology that would be used by staff in Region H and Region S. Here, patients could attend their appointments through an online dedicated private portal from the digital service provider MyChart, a dedicated EPIC app for patients (Region H, 2020). The technology was similar in its function to familiar video conference systems, but it also ensured encryption and privacy between patient and doctor. Healthcare staff and their patients adapted to the service relatively quickly as a result of implementation initiatives. 'Department *champions*' (nurses, doctors, or clinical secretaries) were appointed as implementation partners to promote the technology and encourage its use. They were also encouraged to (a) refer to and communicate the technology, (b) be responsible for staff adoption, and (c) lead the department-level adoption of the video consultancy tool.

A report conducted by Region H showed a "dramatic" uptake in the number of video consultations in the period after COVID-19 had emerged. This report illustrated the uptake of video consultations during Denmark's first two waves of COVID-19 in the spring and winter of 2020 (Region H, 2020).

The video consultation feature was available for use by all clinical staff with patient contact after the first wave of the pandemic. Region H announced that the video consultation feature would remain after COVID-19 as a permanent digital option within the information infrastructure.

Contact tracing: New add-on solution based on existing data structures in the installed base

Many of the needs that had emerged during the opening stages of COVID-19 could be met by enabling, utilising or reconfiguring existing digital solutions. This enabled urgent digital change to take place by extending the installed base. Pre-COVID-19, this had been handled through a plan-driven (and time-consuming) approach whereby new features were carefully developed and tested before being introduced to a wide audience. The COVID-19 crisis period required a new type of digital vigilance through which novel solutions were either developed or acquired and implemented, tested, and potentially reconfigured quickly by taking a highly agile approach.

An example of this came during the first wave of COVID-19, in 2020, when EPIC released a new tool for contact tracing of patients and staff to prevent the potential spread of the COVID-19 virus (CIMT, 2021). Contact tracing was important, as patients could be allocated and moved between wards and healthcare staff shifts while they had COVID-19 (whether having tested positive or not), thus risking spreading the virus among staff and between wards.

The new contact tracing tool was initially offered as a standard solution from the EPIC vendor based on the existing data structures in the EPIC database. To enable the rapid and satisfactory implementation of the tool, a task group was established that consisted of clinicians, IT staff and heads of department. This task force translated the tool (from English to Danish) and made technical configurations to meet the Danish context, including querying and extracting relevant patient data from the regions' EPIC-based EHR system. Within just two weeks, the tool was configured and tested on a small user group in a limited organisational setting. Based on these tests, the tool was deemed ready for large-scale implementation in hospitals. It was possible to complete this urgent digital change across all hospitals because the contact tracing feature was generic across all clinical areas.

The contact tracing generated three types of report. The first was to summarise COVID-19-positive patients who were currently admitted or had been discharged within the previous five days. The second was to provide an overview of the rooms in which a COVID-19-positive patient had been located during admission and in the previous three days. The third was to show which patients had been physically present in the same room during the previous three days.

The health professionals' responses were initially positive, since the automated contact tracing worked efficiently and saved them significant time, as they would otherwise have had to manually trace patients by looking up information in their medical records. One nurse stated: 'It is easy to work with, and it saves a lot of time. Previously we had to look up each patient and would spend half a day on contact tracing for just one patient. Now it can be done in half an hour'.

Limiting the time for contact tracing from hours to minutes led to extensive use of the tool. From 26 April 2020, until the end of June 2020, the tool was used for 3755 contact tracings (Source: Region H, internal communication).

Configuring COVID-19 illness trajectories: Introducing additional data entry and data structures to the installed base

When diseases such as COVID-19 with unknown illness trajectories and uncertain risk profiles for public health spread in society, best practices can be difficult to achieve and maintain in a standard manner across all healthcare staff and clinical domains. Patients would therefore be at risk of receiving non-standard treatment plans from well-meaning doctors trying to act upon real-life illness symptoms as they occurred in an escalating manner. This would, in turn, increase the risk of patients contracting such diseases.

EPIC offers so-called 'clinical order sets' as a functionality to support standard treatment plans. Digital clinical order sets are pre-built, structured templates that are known to help senior clinicians and experts in creating standard treatment plans (including medicine, examinations, observations, etc.) and rolling them out to colleagues in local departments or sharing them across clinical domains as region-wide standard treatment packages. Clinical order sets are customisable and can be tailored to the specific needs and workflows of individual healthcare organisations. They also have the capacity to be updated in real time.

A task force was established to work in collaboration with national experts that gathered global evidence to inform the appropriate order sets to be used across the hospitals in both regions. Order sets with treatment plans were made available to all clinical staff who treated COVID-19 patients, enabling the ongoing distribution of procedures aligned with the most recent knowledge and best practices.

The pressing need to technically configure the EPIC-based EHR system to clearly communicate vast amounts of information to clinicians and to support the distributed order sets was a great challenge for the task force. It was a complex and difficult task to configure the underlying data structure of the EHR database, especially since new and relevant knowledge of the disease was continuously emerging. Clinics across both regions would rapidly provide crucial feedback for the task force, including asking for new adjustments to the order sets and the underlying data structure, since the increasing number of COVID-19 patients provided more local knowledge.

The task force experienced delays and issues when clinicians requested configurations through a distributed network of regional IT personnel. The IT organisation struggled to manage development processes and ensure a continuous dialogue with clinicians. The following five factors, at least, critically challenged the rapid response in the development, adjustment, and maintenance of the order sets:

1 The need to continuously follow up on changing guidelines: COVID-19 was a new disease, and the guidelines for its management changed rapidly both nationally and internationally. This made it difficult to keep order sets up to date.
2 Variability of the severity of COVID-19: the disease exhibited a wide range of symptoms and levels of severity that made it difficult to develop one-size-fits-all order sets. Order sets needed to be able to handle great variability due to the long-term effects of the disease and the fact that the efficacy of the different treatments was unknown.
3 COVID-19 introduced new clinical concepts and classifications: new database tables and data entry had to be defined in the EHR system to encompass such a completely new disease as COVID-19. Normally, changes to the database structure would require thorough analysis because they would affect other data structures and functionalities of the EHR system.
4 Limited technical resources: COVID-19 put a strain on a healthcare system with limited IT development resources. The technical configuration of the EHR database (the heart of the information infrastructure) was complex and required highly specialised developers. The task force faced an IT organisation pushed to the limits of its capabilities and unable to undertake an agile approach with successive region-wide or local iterations.

5 Failure of feedback procedures: procedures for providing critical user feedback and change requests had been developed to facilitate a six-month release cycle, but they broke down during spring 2020. The need for urgent iterations and continuous requests for iterations and local reconfigurations were in many cases not addressed.

During the implementation of new order sets for COVID-19, clinicians experienced disruptions to their workflow, which had implications for other clinical workflows. Testing the digital changes before roll-out was underprioritised, and as a result, clinicians across clinical domains experienced uncertainty about when a patient had been diagnosed and for how long after a diagnosis the patient should remain on the order set recommendations. In some cases, patients were still flagged as having COVID-19 more than three weeks after their preliminary diagnosis, leading to concerns about the validity of the system's ability to provide timely information to clinicians. The task force was criticised for not being able to handle end-user feedback in a structured way. Slow, disrupted or ignored responses to clinical feedback resulted in clinical staff experiencing frustration. This initiated a debate over whether doctors should be granted autonomy to avoid the consequences of misunderstandings in the EHR system's workflow, for example by accepting exceptions to the standard to honour primary care purposes. For a long time, doctors could not rely on the system's indicators of patients during their incubation periods, which severely hampered individual patient treatment as well as the planning and coordination of patient care trajectories.

Discussion

In the following, we summarise the three cases by outlining their distinct characteristics. Then we assess the implications of maintaining digital vigilance to meet future needs for urgent digital change, which are summarised in Table 9.1.

Video consultancy had been introduced into the Danish healthcare sector prior to COVID-19, albeit with mixed results (Folker et. al., 2018; Wentzer, 2013), and there was resistance among healthcare staff, who anecdotally preferred and demanded to see and examine their patients physically (Catapan & Calvo, 2020). Most hospital staff insisted on the personal attendance of patients in hospitals as the dominant standard procedure for all diagnostics and treatments. A pre-COVID report compiled by Region H based on 22 patient interviews (Region H, 2020) concluded that while the video consultancy feature could help many patients, the ability of patients and doctors to choose for themselves was still recommended. This changed dramatically during COVID-19, when video consultancy was rapidly and broadly adopted.

The video consultancy technology case represented a dormant solution (i.e., an inactive or rarely used digital solution) pre-existing in the installed base.

Table 9.1 Implications of maintaining digital vigilance to meet future needs for urgent digital change, summarised as solution strategy, consideration, and vigilance exemplified by the three cases

Solution strategy – example case	*Consideration*	*Vigilance*
Adaptation of dormant digital solutions from the installed base • Video consultation	Do we have a solution 'in stock' in our installed base that we can activate?	• Good overview of latent digital solutions that meet standards and safety requirements • Capability to roll out quickly • Support for all users • Documentation in place and tested
New add-on solutions based on existing data structures in the installed base • Contact tracing	Can we procure or develop a solution that can quickly and smoothly be imported into our installed base?	• Good overview of existing data, data structures, and functionalities • Rapid development capability aligned with clinical procedures • Capability to pilot, implement, and evaluate prior to roll-out
Introducing additional data entry and data structures to the installed base • Configuring COVID-19 illness trajectories	Can we quickly develop and evaluate a solution and maintain continuous iterations and local reconfigurations to meet emergent change needs?	• Agile participatory design and development capability aligned with clinical needs, procedures, and practices • Capability to pilot, implement, and evaluate prior to roll-out • Efficient feedback structure to capture emergent needs for reconfiguration • Capability to engage in continuous iterations and distributed local reconfiguration efforts

This feature was part of Region H's portfolio of available ready-to-use tools, i.e., it was a tool that satisfied the required standards (including safety and privacy requirements) and had the necessary documentation, user guides, support organisation, etc., in place. Video consultancy was a technology familiar to clinicians and most patients. Furthermore, it functioned as an autonomous solution (i.e., a self-contained 'stand-alone' solution) that could be used independently of other technologies.

The contact tracing case outlined the need for a digital solution that did not exist prior to COVID-19. Contact tracing was developed as an extension to the EPIC system based on a new standard tool developed and provided by the vendor. This tool was relatively easy to configure to accommodate the regions' EHR systems and regional/national procedures. Basically, the contact tracing was a report facility that generated three types of lists of clinicians and patients who had a potential risk of being infected. These contact tracing reports could be extracted and generated from the existing data available in the EHR system, leaving other data structures and functionalities in the installed base unaffected. The use of contact tracing was generic across all medical units, and the initial testing of this new digital solution could be done in isolation by a subset of medical units involving a relatively small selection of clinicians. In this way, the evaluation of the contact tracing and the accompanying need for documentation, guidelines and support could be determined during one or several iterations before the solution was made available to the entire organisation. Contact tracing could be performed by dedicated clinicians as a new autonomous task independent of other clinical workflows integrated with patient trajectories.

Video consultancy and contact tracing represent two technologies that, while not unproblematic, saw rapid implementation success by not requiring complex integration with local clinical workflows, and the perspectives of both examples were by their nature relevant across specialities. Such tools provide an example of a quick and successful implementation that was driven by urgent needs and show that such implementations can be carried out successfully when the stakeholders in question collaborate with clinical staff. Furthermore, the cases have shown a potential for permanent and more extensive usage, possibly after local adaptation, to meet the needs of other areas within the healthcare sector.

The case of configuring COVID-19 illness trajectories demonstrates configuration as an embedded change of the installed base to meet new needs. Developing new order sets supporting clinical workflows for COVID-19-related patient trajectories involved the introduction of new clinical concepts, classifications, and diagnoses to document a completely new course of disease. Technically, this implied introducing additional data structures and data entry embedded in the installed base (i.e. changes to the central EHR database). In contrast to video consultancy and contact tracing, the order sets and workflows for COVID-19 patients were meticulously integrated with clinicians' documentation of patient trajectories. The initial implementation focused on documenting and monitoring the spread of the disease and was immediately accepted and applied by clinicians who received patients hospitalised with COVID-19. However, problems soon arose when the COVID-19 patient trajectories evolved, when the clinicians faced an overwhelming amount of information and guidelines and when unanticipated complexities emerged, e.g., when COVID-19 patients had passed the incubation period while still hospitalised for other reasons. Clinicians from different clinical specialities continuously reported problems and the need for changes, but these requests were not properly addressed. The organisation was not prepared for or capable of meeting the user feedback, emergent change requests, and the need for continuous iterations and local reconfigurations. The case demonstrates more extensive implications and a need for local adaptation that was not allowed or met by centrally governed digital changes. As a heavily sociotechnical embedded change, this led to the requirement for greater sensitivity to speciality needs, a need for an iterative approach to the ongoing implementation and the possibility of making local configurations. We noted that this digital change had received a rough start due to its strong need for documentation, local adaptation, the technological re-education of staff, and strict guidelines that were poorly supported locally. Feedback from users was not properly addressed, and the command line of feedback from users was not clear to clinical staff.

The three cases clearly illustrate situations whereby a routine, plan-driven, and release-based approach to digital change falls short. From these cases, we can elicit some general implications such as initial guidelines to establish vigilance in order to meet future urgent digital change needs. An urgent change implies readiness for an agile development and implementation trajectory to bring project time and closure to a head.

The video consultation case represents a solution strategy that might be a feasible first-choice approach if it could meet the change needed. It requires the organisation to have a relevant digital solution ready as part of the portfolio of applications in the installed base. The necessary support facilities and resources, as well as the required documentation, must be present or able to swiftly be established. If no relevant solution is 'in stock', the next logical consideration might be to acquire a new digital solution to be added to the installed base as an add-on. The contact tracing case represents a solution that utilises existing data and functionality and provides the necessary information and functionality without compromising or changing the EHR facilities used in the ordinary clinical processes and patient trajectories. As a general solution, it could be configured, documented, and evaluated by a small subset of users as a pilot implementation (Hertzum et al., 2012) before being rolled out to all clinicians. Finally, it might be necessary to develop new EHR functionality embedded as part of the installed base, illustrated in the case of configuring COVID-19 illness trajectories. This solution strategy is ambitious but risky and includes changes to the everyday practice of managing and documenting patient trajectories through the EHR system. It also includes configurations that alter or introduce new classification systems, data entry, and functionality that need to be adapted to clinical work practices. It is very difficult, or indeed impossible, to anticipate all the consequences of introducing such changes, since the solution needs to be closely integrated with both the technology (EHR) and the work procedures and practices affected. Vigilance in this case implies capabilities for sustained iterations and options for local configuration (Simonsen & Hertzum, 2012, 2022).

Conclusion

As we have shown in this chapter, COVID-19 required an urgent transition in the healthcare sector, not only regarding clinical practices and procedures but also within the information infrastructures that enabled an efficient response to this health crisis. Before COVID-19, digital change typically took place as part of lengthy processes through which new solutions were carefully developed and tested before implementation. However, as we found in this study, the COVID-19 pandemic required human, organisational, and technological resources to be mobilised in unprecedented ways to quickly develop efficient support for healthcare staff in diagnosing, tracing, and treating patients infected with the new virus.

We labelled our empirical findings as digital vigilance to describe the human, organisational, and technological factors required for establishing an effective digital crisis response and the processes required to mobilise these. Based on our findings, we identified and characterised three variants of digital vigilance that took place during COVID-19.

Limitations and comment on research ethics

Our findings are relevant for hospitals that are seeking to learn about the implications of digital contingency during events requiring swift transitions. The findings are derived from a modern hospital system with a centralised governance structure where high levels of standardisation are among the main obstacles to rapid or local transitions. Furthermore, the findings are primarily relevant for hospitals and healthcare decision-makers that operate in highly digital settings, such as cross-hospital healthcare information systems and EHR systems. Our analysis and communication of the empirical cases were on a distanced and general level and thus in accordance with research ethics guidelines within this field.

Note

1 www.epic.com. In Danish, *Sundhedsplatformen* (www.regionh.dk//sundhedsplatformen; www.regionsjaelland.dk/sundhedsplatformen).

References

Aanestad, M., Grisot, M., Hanseth, O., & Vassilakopoulou, P. (2017). Information infrastructures and the challenge of the installed base. In M. Aanestad, M. Grisot, O. Hanseth, & P. Vassilakopoulou (Eds.), *Information infrastructures within European health care: Working with the installed base*. Springer. 10.1007/978-3-319-51020-0

Bansler, J. P. (2019). Adaptation of clinical information infrastructures by and for users. *Infrahealth 2019 – Proceedings of the 7th International Workshop on Infrastructure in Healthcare 2019*. European Society for Socially Embedded Technologies (EUSSET). https://dl.eusset.eu/bitstream/20.500.12015/3312/1/INFRAHEALTH_2019_paper_1.pdf

Bansler, J. P. (2021). Challenges in user-driven optimization of EHR: A case study of a large Epic implementation in Denmark. *International Journal of Medical Informatics, 148.* 10.1016/j.ijmedinf.2021.104394

Barasa, E., Mbau, R., & Gilson, L. (2018). What is resilience and how can it be nurtured? A systematic review of empirical literature on organizational resilience. *International Journal of Health Policy Management*, *7*(6), 491–503. 10.15171/ijhpm.2018.06

Baskerville, R., & Pries-Heje, J. (2021). Achieving resilience through agility. *ICIS 2021 Proceedings, 8.* https://aisel.aisnet.org/icis2021/is_resilience/is_resilience/8/

Bhamra, R., Dani, S., & Burnard, K. (2011). Resilience: The concept, a literature review and future directions. *International Journal of Production Research, 49*(18), 5375–5393. 10.1080/00207543.2011.563826

Catapan, S. D C., & Calvo, M. C. M. (2020). Teleconsultation: An integrative review of the doctor-patient interaction mediated by technology.. *Revista Brasileira de Educação Médica, 44.*

CIMT (2021). *SP-statusrapport April 2021* [EPIC status report, April 2021] Center for IT og Medicoteknologi, Copenhagen.

Folker, M. P., Helverskov, T., Nielsen, A. S., Jørgensen, U. S., & Larsen, J. T. (2018). Telepsykiatri giver nye muligheder for forebyggelse og behandling af psykisk sygdom. *Ugeskrift for Læger, 180*, V07170572.

Hanseth, O., & Lyytinen, K. (2010). Design theory for dynamic complexity in information infrastructures: The case of building internet. *Journal of Information Technology, 25*(1), 1–19. 10.1057/jit.2009.19

Herbig, P. A., & Kramer, H. (1993). Innovation inertia: The power of the installed base. *Journal of Business & Industrial Marketing, 8*(3), 44–57. 10.1108/08858629310044165

Hertzum, M., Bansler, J. P., Havn, E. C., & Simonsen, J. (2012). Pilot implementation: Learning from field tests in IS development. *Communications of the Association for Information Systems, 30*(1), 313–328. 10.17705/1CAIS.03020

Karasti, H., Baker, K. S., & Millerand, F. (2010). Infrastructure time: Long-term matters in collaborative development. *Computer Supported Cooperative Work, 19*(3–4), 377–415. 10.1007/s10606-010-9113-z

Kitamura, C., Zurawel-Balaura, L., & Wong, R. K. S. (2010). How effective Is video consultation in clinical oncology? A systematic review. *Current Oncology, 17*(3), 17–27. 10.3747/co.v17i3.513

Region, H. (2020). *Videokonsultationer via MinSP - et godt alternativ til fremmøde* [Video consultations via MyChart – a good alternative to physical attendance]. Capital Region of Denmark. https://www.regionh.dk/patientinddragelse/udgivelser/udgivelser/Documents/Rapport_Patientoplevet%20kvalitet%20ved%20videokonsultationer%20i%20MinSP.pdf

Simonsen, J., & Hertzum, M. (2012). Sustained participatory design: Extending the iterative approach. *Design Issues, 28*(3), 10–21. 10.1162/DESI_a_00158

Simonsen, J., & Hertzum, M. (2022). Effects-driven IT improvement: Pursuing local post-implementation opportunities. *Scandinavian Journal of Information Systems, 34*(1), 37–70. https://aisel.aisnet.org/sjis/vol34/iss1/2/

Stommel, W., Goor, H. V., & Stommel, M. (2019). Other-attentiveness in video consultation openings: A conversation analysis of video-mediated versus face-to-face consultations. *Journal of Computer-Mediated Communication, 24*(6), 275–292. 10.1093/jcmc/zmz015

Sturt, J., Huxley, C., Ajana, B., Gainty, C., Gibbons, C., Graham, T., Khadjesari, Z., Lucivero, F., Rogers, R., Smol, A., Watkins, J. A., & Griffiths, F. (2020). How does the use of digital consulting change the meaning of being a patient and/or a health professional? Lessons from the Long-term Conditions Young People Networked Communication study. *Digital Health*, *6*, 1–13. 10.1177/2055207620942

Vogus, T. J., & Sutcliffe, K. M. (2007). Organizational resilience: Towards a theory and research agenda. *Proceedings of the IEEE International Conference on Systems Management and Cybernetics*. 10.1109/ICSMC.2007.4414160

Wentzer, H. (2013). Opfølgende hjemmebesøg med video: Et telemedicinsk eksperiment til innovation af tværsektorielt samarbejde [Follow-up home visits with video: A telemedical experiment for innovation in cross-sectoral colloboration]. *KORA*. http://www.kora.dk/media/1220/dsi-3446.pdf

10 COVID-19 in the meat industry

Health and sustainable development in the food sector?

Erling Jelsøe

Introduction

Soon after COVID-19 proliferated outside China in the first half of 2020, outbreaks of infections occurred among slaughterhouse workers across the world, particularly in Europe, the United States, and South America. Many cases involved migrant workers living in poor, cramped housing. Furthermore, it became clear that working conditions in the meat industry carried a great risk of spreading the virus. The outbreaks drew attention to a production sector based on low-paid labour and bad working conditions. This is not in itself something new. Working conditions and recruitment of low-paid labour in the meat industry have been reported on and critically discussed numerous times and have been a familiar feature of the industry in many countries for several decades (see, e.g., Eisnitz, 2007; Haedicke, 2020; Nierenberg, 2005). Added to the low temperatures and poor ventilation typical of slaughterhouses, and workers standing close together, an environment was created that was almost ideal for COVID-19 infection.

These conditions had a negative effect on workers' health, but meat production globally is associated with various other health issues. Excessive use of antibiotics in livestock farming is a source of antimicrobial resistance in pathogenic bacteria. Other pathogens are spreading, particularly in large factory farms, and the intensification of processes in meat plants means that they are transferred to meat products, threatening consumers with infection. Avian flu and swine flu are also spread through intensive livestock farming. These and other disease risks are all connected to how meat is produced in modern large-scale intensified production systems (Nierenberg, 2005; Steinfeld et al., 2006; Weis, 2014).

Furthermore, meat production globally has been increasing. The greatest rise has occurred in China but there has been growth in Europe, the United States and especially in Brazil. Since the early 1960s, there has been an almost fivefold increase in global meat production (Ritchi & Roser, 2019), partly because of the increase in world population but even more due to higher meat consumption per capita, although meat consumption is still very unevenly distributed among countries and regions worldwide. The growth in

DOI: 10.4324/9781003441915-13

meat production is unsustainable in a wider sense than merely in relation to health (Nierenberg, 2005; Weis, 2014). It has been associated with an enormous drain on resources in terms of water, energy, and land. Increasing meat production is an important contributor to climate change. Many experts fear that the clearing of land for agricultural production in itself can increase the risk of spread of diseases and the emergence of future pandemics, because the reduction in habitats for wild animals that carry infectious diseases brings these animals closer to humans and domestic animals.

Seen in this light, COVID-19 is an element in a much larger complex of problems associated with meat production in the modern industrialised food system. Although specific physical and biological factors in meat processing increase the risk of spreading COVID-19 in slaughterhouses, it is the broader socio-economic characteristics of the meat industry that have shaped the processes. The following analyses of the events in selected countries will show that the history of the meat industry in each country has been crucial for the way outbreaks of COVID-19 have unfolded, and the implications for the health of workers and local communities. This particularly involves the utilisation and recruitment of the workforce, the organisation of production, the regulatory history of the industry and the structure and dynamics of the meat supply chains as a whole. It is a history of how the meat industry globally has been able to supply the world market with cheap meat. In their account of the implications of the subcontracting systems in Germany, Solomon et al. (2021) frame the consequences of this development as 'the human costs of cheap meat'. These costs can be seen as the immediate outcome of the subcontracting system, but must also be understood as results of underlying social, political, and economic drivers of the development of the meat supply chain that have enabled large-scale production of cheap meat with all its wider implications for the sustainability of meat production (Nierenberg, 2005; Weis, 2014). The costs of cheap meat are thus also costs for nature and the environment, food safety, and animal welfare. This demonstrates how the social and environmental aspects of sustainable development are connected and how workers' health can be seen in the context of the sustainability of meat production in general.

This chapter will focus on the outbreaks of COVID-19 in slaughterhouses in the context of the historical development of slaughterhouses, with an emphasis on developments in selected countries, particularly the countries with the most pronounced problems, i.e. Germany, the United States, and Brazil. Denmark is included as a country with a somewhat different situation, but which also illustrates the impact of German developments on neighbouring countries. Following this more detailed account of developments, some reflections on the broader context and the complex of unsustainable characteristics of meat production are added to contribute to a discussion about a transition towards more sustainable food systems.

Sustainable development: Some conceptual remarks

Since this chapter focuses on the sustainability of food production, a brief clarification of the concept of sustainability and its relation to health is pertinent. As pointed out by several authors (e.g. Langhelle, 2002; Redclift, 1987; Weis, 2014), the concept of sustainable development as introduced by the Brundtland Commission in 1987 (World Commission on Environment and Development, 1987) is contradictory in not resolving the conflict between environmental and social problems (e.g. social inequality, excessive resource utilisation, and destruction of habitats) and the patterns of economic growth and the dynamics and power relations that have created these problems. The global development of the food system illustrates these conflicts, which will be discussed further in this chapter.

The virtue of the concept of sustainable development is its focus on people's needs and its interaction with environmental issues. The concept is represented as a holistic whole of three pillars: environmental, social, and economic sustainability. The normative understanding of development as a means for achieving social goals through societal change is well expressed by Kickbusch (2010, p. 8): 'sustainable development implies a paradigm shift from a model of development based on inequity and exploitation of resources to one that requires new forms of responsibility, solidarity and accountability not only on the national but also on the global level'.

The social dimension has often been deprioritised in understandings of sustainable development, despite being crucial in the sense that human agency in relation to the economy and the environment is always embedded in and conditioned by social contexts (Dillard et al., 2009; Jelsøe et al., 2018; Parra, 2013). Thus, health as an aspect of the concept of sustainable development is fundamentally related to social sustainability. For instance, working and living conditions of the workforce in slaughterhouses and their implications for workers' health must be understood in terms of the social sustainability (or lack of it) of slaughterhouse production. However, these conditions are also expressions of environmental and material factors in the production sector and therefore related to environmental sustainability. This holistic understanding of health as related to social, environmental, and economic sustainability has been expressed as a socio-ecological perspective on health (Dooris, 1999; Kickbusch, 2010).

The relevance of the socio-ecological perspective on health becomes even more pertinent if one considers the health aspects of the food supply chain as a whole. The broad range of health issues connected with the modern food system as outlined above is related to the ways in which the natural environment and biological resources have been subordinated to the dynamics of capitalist production. The historical development of food production, or what might be termed the capitalist transformation of food production, has led to comprehensive changes in all links of the supply chain, both technologically and structurally. These changes have created new health and environmental risks for employees in the food sector.

Data and methods

None of the countries studied here have official data on outbreaks of COVID-19 or the number of workers infected. These data have been obtained from various alternative sources. Statistics on the number of infected workers and on outbreaks in the various countries were primarily found in reports from various organisations and information networks such as EFFAT (the European Federation of Food, Agriculture and Tourism Trade Unions) and, in the United States, the FERN (Food and Environment Reporting Network), and the Select Committee on the Coronavirus Crisis of the US Congress. In the United States, the Center for Disease Control and Prevention (CDC) also published data from some states that had reported on outbreaks of COVID-19 in the meat industry. In Brazil, there were no systematic accounts of outbreaks or numbers of people infected, but local health authorities reported outbreaks in some of the states.

Outbreaks were covered extensively in the media in all affected countries. Media sources and data were obtained through searches in Google and Google Scholar using the search words 'slaughterhouse/meat industry/ meatpacker AND COVID-19/corona'. In some searches, a country prefix was added. The word 'outbreaks' together with COVID-19 was also used. In searches for sources regarding labour market conditions, the words 'labour/ labor market' and/or 'migrants/migrant workers' were added. Some sources for Brazil were references written in Portuguese and were translated into Danish and English using Google Translate. As far as possible, media articles and reports were taken from recognised sources such as *The Washington Post* and *The Guardian* and news agencies such as Reuters and Bloomberg News.

This chapter was written shortly after the outbreaks took place, and there were thus quite few scientific publications analysing them. The scientific publications included as sources were found via searches on Google Scholar using the same search words as mentioned above. In searches for historical analyses of developments in the meat industry, the words 'COVID-19/ corona' were omitted.

Rationale for the choice of the selected countries

The selected countries were chosen partly because they had the most pronounced problems with COVID-19 in slaughterhouses, as judged from existing accounts. Further, Germany, the United States, and Brazil are among the largest meat producers in the world. Nevertheless, problems with COVID-19 in slaughterhouses occurred in countries all over the world, with similar issues to those in the three countries studied (for Europe, see EFFAT, 2020). Therefore, despite variations in specific developments between countries, the selected countries can illuminate more general causes and drivers for developments in most other countries.

COVID-19 in the meat industry

Figures for the total number of workers infected in slaughterhouses and meat processing plants in the various countries are notoriously difficult to obtain. One reason is that meat producers have often been disinclined to release such information (see, e.g., Douglas, 2020). Numbers of infected workers have thus been part of the social and political controversy around the outbreaks. Findings from the United States indicate that more than 59 000 workers were infected and at least 298 died from March 2020 until 2 September 2021 (Douglas, 2021; US Congress, 2021). In Brazil, an estimate by the national workers' union suggests that one in five workers in Brazil's meat plants was infected, which equates to over 100 000 of the country's half a million workers. Although this estimate was rejected by representatives of the industry, other reports suggest many thousands of cases at many meat plants (Freitas, 2020; Garcia et al., 2022; Mano, 2020a; Pina, 2020; Segata et al., 2021). According to estimates from the Food, Beverages and Catering Union in Germany, about 30 000–35 000 or one-third of meat industry workers were infected (Staunton, 2021).

Germany

As mentioned above, there are no official estimates of the total number of infected workers in German slaughterhouses. Early outbreaks were reported in the first half of April 2020 (Finci et al., 2022; Romania Insider, 2020), but during the spring and summer 2020 many outbreaks took place across Germany (EFFAT, 2020; Pokora et al., 2021). May saw a major outbreak at a slaughterhouse owned by Westfleisch, the second largest meat company in Germany, in North Rhine-Westphalia, which led the state to activate an 'emergency brake', which meant delaying the relaxing of lockdown restrictions in the administrative district. The plant was also shut down (EFFAT, 2020; Jordans, 2020).

The biggest and most significant outbreak in Germany was in Reda-Wiedenbrück in the largest pig slaughterhouse in the country, also in North Rhine-Westphalia, in June 2020. At the plant, owned by Tönnies, by far the largest meat processing company in Germany, more than 1500 of 7000 employees tested positive. The plant was shut down for a month and all positive cases of workers, their relatives, and those with whom they shared accommodation, totalling over 6500 people, were quarantined. Furthermore, because of the risk of infecting the communities around the plant, lockdown restrictions applied in the earlier phases of COVID-19 in Germany were re-introduced in the surrounding districts, thus affecting all inhabitants in the area (Buch, 2020; EFFAT, 2020; Markvardsen, 2020).

There were lockdowns at several other slaughterhouses in Germany and outbreaks at many more. The German health authorities issued recommendations for work during COVID-19 that included distancing, face coverings, personal protective equipment, cleaning, and hand hygiene (Pokora et al., 2021). However, meat processing companies were criticised for not implementing the measures or only doing so inadequately and too late (EFFAT, 2020). It was also pointed out that in several cases, including the ones mentioned above, they were reluctant to close down the plants when infections among workers proliferated. There was also criticism of insufficient inspection by the authorities regarding violations of health and safety measures during the pandemic.

The outbreaks of COVID-19 drew attention to working conditions in the slaughterhouses. These involved labour-intensive repetitive processes at a high pace, with physical and mental stress, and frequent injuries. Furthermore, workers stand almost shoulder to shoulder in cold rooms, where the virus is transmitted more easily. Several studies also demonstrated that air circulation and lack of ventilation increased the risk of infection and especially the distance over which infections could be transmitted (Finci et al., 2022; Günther et al., 2020; Pokora et al., 2021).

Above all, COVID-19 drew renewed attention to the particular work and housing conditions of meat industry workers. The most important work processes are mostly performed by migrant workers from Central and Eastern Europe, primarily from Bulgaria, Poland, and Romania, who are employed by subcontractors. They receive very low wages and often live in overcrowded accommodation that they rent from the subcontractor. The general housing and transport conditions involve a considerable risk of infection.

Although German legislation from 2015 states that workers should be employed by German companies and meet German labour market rules, including the German minimum wage (9.35 euro per hour in 2020), migrant workers often receive lower wages, with long working hours and unpaid overtime. The meat companies are not responsible for these conditions, because the responsibility is handed over to the subcontractors. Furthermore, ill workers are often afraid of staying away from work, because of the fear of losing their job, and may not receive paid sick leave (for more detailed accounts of the subcontracting system and its consequences, see, e.g., Solomon et al., 2021; Wagner & Hassel, 2016; Whittail & Trinczek, 2020).

Assessments of the number of workers employed by subcontractors vary somewhat, but one estimate is that this applies to around 30 000 workers out of a total workforce in the German meat industry of approximately 110 000. In the big meat companies, however, the percentage of workers employed by subcontractors is estimated at around 80–90% (EFFAT, 2020).

Criticism of the subcontracting system in Germany was not new during COVID-19, but the outbreaks fuelled the debate and fostered a political initiative. In December 2020, the German Bundestag passed a new act, the Occupational Health and Safety Control Act, which prohibited subcontracting in the meat industry. Meat companies had to employ workers directly themselves. The act introduced electronic recording of working hours and a minimum rate of workplace inspections to prevent long and unpaid working hours. Violations of the rules can lead to fines of up to EUR

30 000. This act, which came in force almost immediately in 2021, is seen as a breakthrough for the opposition to the subcontracting system.

However, there is still some concern about whether the act will put an end to the problems. Experience from the political intervention in 2015, where the previous so-called posting system was abandoned, was negative (Ban et al., 2022; Staunton, 2021).

Other countries beside Germany use subcontracting in the meat industry. In many other European countries, subcontracting functions in various ways (EFFAT, 2020; McSweeny & Young, 2021). Following the German legislation, members of the European Parliament attempted to introduce a ban on subcontracting in the meat industry in the European Union as a whole (Rankin, 2021). Subcontracting in various forms had existed in Germany since the late 1980s and escalated during the 1990s and 2000s, when the German meat industry became very competitive, and German pork production in particular rose by almost 50% (Simons & Lenders, 2020; Whittail & Trinczek, 2020).

These developments have had repercussions throughout the meat supply chain. Cheap meat has been available and big supermarket chains have used their market power to put pressure on meat prices. Solomon et al. (2021), in discussing the human consequences of the subcontracting system, refer to 'the human cost of cheap meat'. The human cost is evident for the workers, both generally as a result of the subcontracting system and more specifically in relation to the COVID-19 pandemic in slaughterhouses. In addition, however, there is a cost in a wider sense regarding the sustainability of the food system due to the rapid, unsustainable growth of meat production.

Denmark

When COVID-19 started in spring 2020, no problems were reported in Danish slaughterhouses. Unlike Germany, all Danish and foreign workers receive wages based on collective agreements, and wages are much higher than in Germany. Around 35% of the workers are migrants and are employed on the same conditions as Danish workers. Furthermore, foreign workers have their own accommodation independent of their employers (EFFAT, 2020; Wagner & Refslund, 2016). The slaughterhouses appear to have followed the Danish rules on social distancing, plexiglass barriers between workers, personal protective equipment, etc. (EFFAT, 2020).

Nevertheless, in late July 2020, a significant outbreak occurred in Danish Crown's slaughterhouse in Ringsted, 50 km from Copenhagen. The virus was spreading despite all attempts from the management to contain it, and 160 of about 900 employees became infected. It was then decided to close the plant and the workers had self-isolate. The plant was closed for 12 days and reopened at reduced capacity (Landbrugsavisen, 2020; Tiirikainen & Koch, 2020).

In the search for explanations of the outbreak, attention was drawn to the general risk factors associated with working conditions in slaughterhouses.

There was also a focus on the Polish migrant workers, who lived in cramped conditions, being only temporary workers and wanting to save money. Many also went to work with several people in the same car (Redanz & Rasmussen, 2020).

A different and important aspect of the development in the Danish meat industry was the competitive impact of German developments. From 2001 to 2015, the workforce at Danish Crown, by far the largest slaughterhouse company, was reduced from 16 000 to 8500 at its production facilities in Denmark. In the same period, employment at Danish Crown's facilities in other countries increased from 7300 to 17 500 (Erhardtsen, 2015). One explanation was technological development and large-scale operations in the Danish slaughterhouses. Due to high wages in Denmark, Danish Crown developed its production processes technologically, especially the slaughtering process, to become among the most advanced in the world (Hovgaard, 2021). Some of the more labour-intensive processes like deboning and fine-cutting were moved to factories in other countries, especially Germany. In Germany, Danish Crown used the subcontracting system like the rest of the meat industry (Wagner & Refslund, 2016). Danish Crown is the fourth largest meat company in Germany. The Dutch meat company Vion, the third largest in Germany, has followed a similar strategy. The competitive pressure from low-wage employment in the German subcontracting system has led meat companies in other European countries to practise 'wage dumping' by moving part of their production to Germany.

The United States

In the United States, there were many outbreaks in many slaughterhouses and the problems have been assessed as even greater than in Germany, although comparisons are difficult. Yet there are clear similarities to Germany. In both countries, many workers are migrants (or ethnic minorities in the United States) working at very low wages. The United States has also greatly increased its meat production. From 1990 to 2018, meat production rose by almost 64% (Ritchi & Roser, 2019) and the same period also saw many mergers and centralisation of production plants (Howard, 2019; Huber, 2020).

Working conditions are also generally poor in US slaughterhouses. Production line speeds have been raised to a very high level, and unlike in Europe, they are regulated by the federal government. Further, line speeds are subject to ongoing political debates and controversy, which probably indicates that they are generally higher in the United States, as supported by some observers (Huber, 2020). Several studies indicate that raising line speeds also causes more cases of COVID-19 because workers stand closer together and physical strains are greater (Dorning & Hirtzer, 2020; Kindy et al., 2021; Novic, 2021).

Workplace injuries in the United States have also increased over time. Thus, Krumel (2017) demonstrates how wage levels fell from 1970 to

2010, while the percentages of Hispanic workers and injuries per worker increased considerably (figures for injuries were only until 2000, however). Raising line speeds also causes more injuries (Dorning & Hirtzer, 2020; Novic, 2021).

The first reports of COVID-19 outbreaks in the US meat industry appeared in March 2020 and the number of outbreaks and infections soon proliferated. Many plants closed down for shorter or longer periods, and companies were criticised for being slow to introduce protective measures, testing, and paid sick leave (Laughland & Holpuch, 2020; Lussenhop, 2020; US Congress, 2021). The closures led to decreases in the supply of meat to grocery stores and restaurants and there were reports of lack of meat. On 28 April 2020, Tyson, the largest meat company in the United States, placed full-page advertisements in several leading newspapers, claiming that 'the food supply chain is breaking'. On the following day, President Trump issued an executive order with reference to the Defense Production Act of 1950 to keep meat processing plants open, arguing that meat plants were 'critical infrastructure', crucial to the nation's food supply. Trump's order was widely criticised for not paying sufficient attention to the health and safety of the workers (Boehm, 2020; Telford et al., 2020).

These incidents illustrate different reactions to the COVID-19 crisis in slaughterhouses between the United States and Europe, as exemplified by Germany, where the government reacted in favour of the public good by legislating against subcontracting. In the United States, corporate power and lobbying seemed to influence the government's reaction much more strongly. Further, the Occupational Health and Safety Administration was criticised for not acting effectively in response to the situation. An estimate shows that nearly 90% of all facilities of the five biggest US meat companies had outbreaks with multiple cases of infected workers (Douglas, 2022).

Another significant effect of outbreaks of COVID-19 in slaughterhouses was the spread of infection to the surrounding communities, especially in counties with large production facilities. Studies have revealed that COVID-19 cases in these counties were considerably higher than in comparable counties without slaughterhouses (Krumel & Goodrich, 2021; Taylor et al., 2020).

The fall in meat production reflected the vulnerability of the meat supply chain in the United States, because production was centralised to a limited number of very large plants. If one big plant closed down, it was difficult for farmers to deliver their animals to other slaughterhouses. Furthermore, because many farms are very large with huge numbers of animals, when the slaughterhouses could not receive the animals, millions were culled in spring 2020, leading to challenges in animal welfare and environmental issues connected to the disposal of large numbers of carcasses (Dorning, 2020; Kevany, 2020; Reiley, 2020). The structure of US meat supply chains has led to an unsustainable situation involving a huge waste of resources, environmental problems and animal suffering. Germany also saw a decrease in meat production in 2020, but greater flexibility in German meat supply chains meant that no animals were culled (Simons & Lenders, 2020).

The labour market conditions that provided the context for the COVID-19 outbreaks in the United States, as in Germany, involve a dual labour market and extensive use of migrant workers. The present situation resembles the circumstances in the early 20th century, when Upton Sinclair wrote his famous novel 'The Jungle' about working conditions in the meat industry in Chicago at that time. However, in the first decades after the Second World War, slaughterhouse workers became unionised and gained influence on their wages and working conditions. The unions also worked to overcome discrimination between black and white workers. This changed from the late 1970s, when the meat industry began a restructuring process and moved from industrial areas around big cities like Chicago to small towns in rural areas of the Midwest and South-Eastern US, where there was little tradition of labour unions, and increasingly recruited workers from Mexico and Central America (Haedicke, 2020; Kandel & Parrado, 2005; Krumel, 2017). This is the background to the present situation in the meat industry, where Hispanic workers make up around 45% of the workforce and probably around 15% are Asian (US Congress, 2021, p. 8). These workers are highly vulnerable in crisis situations such as COVID-19. A CDC report on cases of COVID-19 in 23 states found that where race/ethnicity was reported, 87% of cases occurred in racial or ethnic minorities (Waltenburg et al., 2020).

The weakening of labour unions from the 1970s was a feature of the neoliberal period in most Western countries and was also seen in Germany, along with the expansion of the subcontracting system (Whittail & Trinczek, 2020).

Brazil

Together with Germany and the United States, Brazil was probably the country with the most serious problems with COVID-19 outbreaks in slaughterhouses. In Brazil, meat production has increased very considerably during the last 50 years; from 1990 to 2018 it rose by 380% to reach 29.3 million tons, making Brazil one of the four largest meat-producing countries in the world (Ritchi & Roser, 2019). Three of the world's largest meat producers are Brazilian, with JBS currently being the largest in the world.

The number of infected slaughterhouse workers has been disputed in Brazil, but there were reports of outbreaks at many meat plants. The national workers' union estimates that one in five meat industry workers was infected. Most infections occurred in the southern states, but there were also several outbreaks in the western and central parts. In many areas, the outbreaks of COVID-19 at meat plants were reported to be hot spots for spreading the virus to the surrounding communities (Mano, 2020a; Phillips, 2020; Pina, 2020; Segata et al., 2021).

In Brazil, slaughterhouses also used migrant workers extensively, and, in addition, workers from marginalised indigenous communities. Many migrant workers are from Haiti and Venezuela. Haitian workers went to Brazil because of the extreme poverty following the earthquake in Haiti in 2010, and these workers were particularly vulnerable during outbreaks of COVID-19 (Granada, 2021; MercoPress, 2020; Mota, 2020).

Brazilian meat companies were also criticised for being slow to implement preventative measures in slaughterhouses. They were also reluctant to close down factories, even when there were serious outbreaks, and closures often did not take place until special labour courts in Brazil mandated them (Mano, 2020a; Pina, 2020). Two very large multinational meat companies in Brazil, Marfrig and BRF, made agreements with prosecutors in the courts about systematic testing of their workers to avoid more closures, but JBS refused to do this and saw a number of its plants closed by court decisions (Mano, 2020a).

Large Brazilian meat companies also face issues of the sustainability of their operations regarding the use of beef from cattle that has grazed illegally in deforested areas of the Amazon. Brazil has the world's largest number of cattle, and the Amazon region has seen the largest growth in the country's cattle industry. Despite announcements from the companies that they monitor their cattle suppliers thoroughly, they have been unable to convince investors and others that they do not receive cattle from protected areas in the Amazon (Amnesty International, 2020; Mano, 2020b).

Discussion and concluding remarks: Prospects for change in the meat industry

This account of outbreaks of COVID-19 in slaughterhouses has shown how the pandemic unfolded under specific conditions in a production sector with a high risk of spreading the virus. The risk factors are partly related to how production was organised, using biological raw materials of a complex nature, low temperatures, and much manual work. However, the fact that the risk factors resulted in large outbreaks of COVID-19 among workers was also linked to how the meat industry had developed in a broader sense, including the regulatory context, and thus also how companies regulate work processes to maximise income.

There are several common characteristics of the developments in the countries studied. The meat industry in Germany, the United States, and Brazil has a very high pace of work and a production line that practically never stops. Workers' health in all three countries was at risk long before COVID-19 broke out, due to high physical and mental strain and many injuries. Furthermore, the companies in the three countries were slow to introduce protective measures and were disinclined to close production when COVID-19 proliferated in their plants.

The present situation with a high percentage of migrant workers is not incidental but a historical result of the worker recruitment strategies of the meat industry. However, the more specific methods of implementation of these strategies differ between the countries, reflecting different societal conditions. In Germany, the subcontracting system was conditioned by the possibilities for recruitment of cheap labour that arose with the changes in Eastern Europe and the subsequent inclusion of Eastern European countries in the European Union. In the United States, the meat industry underwent a process of relocation and exploited the large numbers of immigrants from Latin America. In Brazil, migrants from countries in the region with huge social problems, particularly Haiti, and poor indigenous people in the country itself were recruited. In Denmark, the most labour-intensive parts of production were moved to Germany, a strategy that has been followed by the meat industry in several other of Germany's neighbouring countries, especially Dutch meat companies.

Common features of the utilisation of migrant workers in the various countries include special housing and transportation conditions, the lack of rights to paid sick leave and the workers' fear of being fired, all of which increased the risk of infection. The labour unions, which were strong in Germany and the United States in the 1970s, were undermined, in Germany through exploitation of the situation following the opening of the labour markets in Eastern Europe and in the United States through relocation of production plants to rural areas and extensive use of migrant workers. The weakening of labour unions has been common to many developed countries in the neoliberal period, but the effects were very pronounced in the meat industry, where it has significantly affected the health and general social conditions of the workers.

Mergers, takeovers, and centralisation of production have led to the establishment of very large production units in both primary production in agriculture and the meat industry, which has made supply chains very fragile in crisis situations such as COVID-19. One consequence was the culling of millions of animals in the United States, which demonstrates the unsustainable development of its meat sector. The very large production plants with thousands of workers also led to large outbreaks of COVID-19 and increased the risk of spreading the virus to the surrounding communities.

The political and regulatory response differed in the countries. Most significant was the German ban on subcontracting. The consequences of the ban are not yet clear; some fear that it may lead to a relocation of parts of the German meat industry to other European countries, notably Spain, where subcontracting is still allowed (Ban et al., 2022). In the United States, the large meat companies put pressure on the federal government, but President Trump's executive order to keep the meat processing plants open had little effect, because many plants had to close down anyway, since the workers fell ill or were afraid to go to work because of the many infected people. Overall, it is still unclear whether the experience of COVID-19 will lead to improvements in any of the countries that would make workers less vulnerable in a new pandemic, or result in any significant changes in working conditions.

The analysis of the outbreaks of COVID-19 in the slaughterhouses and their possible causes point to broader questions of health and sustainability issues related to meat production. They raise the question of transition to a more sustainable and socially just food system. This is not an easy issue to deal with since conditions for transition in the food sector are influenced by strong trajectories of economic and political structures and interests. Much has been written about possible alternatives to the present food systems but the COVID-19 experience adds some points to this.

More generally, Clapp (2020) puts the discussion about a possible transformation of the food system into perspective by discussing the dominant and mainstream suggestions for improvements of the food system versus alternatives put forward by those movements and organisations who challenge the current world food order. Many of the dominant actors in the present food systems advocate a continuation of the existing pattern of development with some improvements, such as technological change, e.g. through sustainable intensification, further intensification of international cooperation through responsible private investment in food production in third world countries, alternatives to the present meat-dominated diets and certification schemes and labelling. The criticism of these measures, however, is that they are often too weak, as in the cases of certification of responsible soybean and palm oil production, and in some instances may even make things worse by increasing the existing market dominance of multinational giants and adding to social inequality.

The COVID-19 crisis has shown how slow the big meat corporations were to implement basic protective measures and how their neglect of adequate employment conditions and exploitation of workers led to serious health and social problems. It is difficult to imagine a future where the meat giants by themselves will offer meat workers socially just and healthy working conditions, unless they are subject to considerable social and political pressure and probably legislation such as the German ban on subcontracting. However, intensification of international trade relations and competitive pressures are likely to make such solutions difficult.

Furthermore, the COVID-19 crisis has shown how unstable and vulnerable to change the meat supply chains are, while developments in recent decades have demonstrated how competitive pressures among big meat companies encourage increased meat production at low prices. The resulting lack of sustainability regarding both social and environmental development suggests a need for more radical change. In a longer-term perspective, this could comprise more resilient solutions, based on the perspectives of a socio-ecological approach, such as community-supported agriculture, more decentralised production units of slaughtering and meat processing and humanisation of working conditions.

References

Amnesty International (2020, July 15, updated October 7). *Brazil: Cattle illegally grazed in the Amazon found in supply chain of leading meat-packer JBS.* Amnesty International. Brazil: Cattle illegally grazed in the Amazon found in supply chain of leading meat-packer JBS (amnesty.org).

Ban, C., Bohle, D., & Naczyk, M. (2022). A perfect storm: COVID-19 and the reorganization of the German meat industry. *Transfer: European Review of Labour and Research, 28*(1), 101–118. 10.1177/10242589221081943

Boehm, R. (2020, May 20). *With Trump executive order, are meat and poultry plants a covid-19 ticking time bomb?* The Equation. Union of Concerned Scientists. With Trump Executive Order, Are Meat and Poultry Plants a COVID-19 Ticking Time Bomb? – Union of Concerned Scientists (ucsusa.org).

Buch, D. (2020, June 23). *Slagteriarbejdere i Tyskland spærret inde efter nyt coronaudbrud* [Slaughterhouse workers in Germany locked up after new COVID-19 outbreak]. TV2. Slagteriarbejdere i Tyskland spærret inde efter nyt coronaudbrud – TV 2.

Clapp, J. (2020). *Food* (3rd ed.). Polity.

Dillard, J., Dujon, V., & King, M. C. (Eds.). (2009). *Understanding the social dimension of sustainability.* Routledge.

Dooris, M. (1999). Healthy cities and local agenda 21: The UK experience – challenges for the new millennium. *Health Promotion International, 14*(4), 365–375. 10.1093/heapro/14.4.365

Dorning, M. (2020, April 28). *America's mass hog cull begins with meat set to rot in landfills.* Bloomberg News. America's Mass Hog Cull Begins with Meat to Rot in Landfills – Bloomberg.

Dorning, M., & Hirtzer, M. (2020, November 11). *Trump makes last push to speed up chicken lines despite pandemic.* Bloomberg News. Trump Makes Last Push to Speed Up Chicken Lines Despite Pandemic – BNN Bloomberg.

Douglas, L. (2020, May 14). *As more meatpacking workers fall ill from Covid-19, meat companies decline to disclose data.* Food & Environment Reporting Network (FERN). As more meatpacking workers fall ill from Covid-19, meat companies decline to disclose data | Food and Environment Reporting Network (thefern.org).

Douglas, L. (2021, September 8). *Mapping COVID-19 outbreaks in the food system.* Food & Environment Reporting Network (FERN). Mapping COVID-19 outbreaks in the food system | Food and Environment Reporting Network (thefern.org).

Douglas, L. (2022, January 14). *Nearly 90% of big US meat plants had COVID-19 cases in pandemic's first year – data.* Reuters. Nearly 90% of big US meat plants had COVID-19 cases in pandemic's first year – data | Reuters.

EFFAT. (2020, June 30). *Covid-19 outbreaks in slaughterhouses and meat processing plants. State of affairs and proposals for policy actions at EU level.* EFFAT Report. European Federation of Food, Agriculture and Tourism Unions (EFFAT). EFFAT-Report-Covid-19-outbreaks-in-slaughterhouses-and-meat-packing-plants-State-of-affairs-and-proposals-for-policy-action-at-EU-level.pdf.

Eisnitz, G. A. (2007). *Slaughterhouse. The shocking story of greed, neglect, and inhumane treatment inside the U.S. meat industry.* Prometheus Books.

Erhardtsen, B. (2015, June 13). *Hver tredje på Danish Crown er udlænding* [Every third worker at Danish Crown is a foreigner]. Berlingske. Hver tredje på Danish Crown er udlænding (berlingske.dk).

Finci, I., Siebenbaum, R., Richtzenhain, J., Edwards, A. Rau, C., Ehrhardt, J., Kolou, L., Joggertst, B., & Brockmann, S. O. (2022). Risk factors associated with an outbreak of COVID-19 in a meat processing plant in Southern Germany, April to June 2020. *Eurosurveillance*, *27*(13), 1–9, 10.2807/1560-7917.ES.2022.27.13.2100354

Freitas, T. (2020, August 19). *Covid hit 20% of meat workers in no. 1 chicken exporter Brazil*. Claims Journal. Covid Hit 20% of Meat Workers in No. 1 Chicken Exporter Brazil (claimsjournal.com).

Garcia, S. D., de Carvalho, M., & Baltazar, M. (2022). Covid-19 among slaughterhouse workers: Relationship between worker's health and food safety. *Revista Brasiliera de Medicina do Trabalho*, *20*(1), 86–93. 10.47626/1679-4435-2022-794

Granada, D. (2021). Health and migration: The COVID-19 pandemic and migrant workers in slaughterhouses in southern Brazil. *Horizontes Antropológicos*, *27*(59), 207–226. 10.1590/s0104-71832021000100011

Günther, T., Czech-Sioli, M., Indenbirken, D., Ribitailles, A., Tenhaken, P., Exner, M. Ottinger, M. Fischner, N., Grubdhof, A., & Brinkmann, M. (2020). Investigation of a superspreading event preceding the largest meat processing plant-related SARS-Coronavirus 2 outbreak in Germany. *EMBO Molecular Medicine*, *12*(12), 1–10. 10.15252/emmm.202013296

Haedicke, M. (2020, May 6). *To understand the danger of COVID-19 outbreaks in meatpacking plants, look at the industry's history*. The Conversation. To understand the danger of COVID-19 outbreaks in meatpacking plants, look at the industry's history (theconversation.com).

Hovgaard, L. (2021, May 18). *Deep learning på slagteriet: Sensorer og algoritmer lærer robotter at føre kniven* [Deep learning in the slaughterhouse. Sensors and algorithms teach robots how to handle the knife]. Ingeniøren. Deep learning på slagteriet: Sensorer og algoritmer lærer robotter at føre kniven | Ingeniøren.

Howard, P. H. (2019). Corporate concentration in global meat processing: The role of feed and finance subsidies. In B. Winders & E. Ransom (Eds.), *Global meat: Social and environmental consequences of the expanding meat industry* (pp. 31–53). MIT Press.

Huber, B. (2020, June 10). *How did Europe avoid the COVID-19 catastrophe ravaging U.S. meatpacking plants?* Food & Environment Reporting Network (FERN). How did Europe avoid the Covid-19 catastrophe ravaging U.S. meatpacking plants? | Food and Environment Reporting Network (thefern.org).

Jelsøe, E., Thualagant, N., Holm, J., Kjærgård, B. Andersen, H. L. M., From, D.-M., Land, B., & Pedersen, K. B. (2018). A future task for health promotion: Integration of health promotion and sustainable development. *Scandinavian Journal of Public Health*, *46*(Suppl. 20), 99–106. 10.1177%2F1403494817744126

Jordans, F. (2020, May 13). *Outbreak at German slaughterhouse reveals migrants plight*. AP News. Outbreak at German slaughterhouse reveals migrants' plight | AP News.

Kandel, W., & Parrado, E. A. (2005). Restructuring of the US meat processing industry and new Hispanic migrant destinations. *Population and Development Review*, *31*(3), 447–471. 10.1111/j.1728-4457.2005.00079.x

Kevany, S. (2020, May 19). *Millions of US farm animals to be culled by suffocation, drowning and shooting*. The Guardian. Millions of US farm animals to be culled by suffocation, drowning and shooting | Environment | The Guardian.

Kickbusch, I. (2010). *Triggering debate – white paper. The food system: A prism of present and future challenges for health promotion and sustainable development.* Health Promotion Switzerland. White-Paper---The-Food-System.pdf (ilona-kickbusch.com).

Kindy, K., Mellnik, T., & Hernandez, A. R. (2021, January 3). The Trump administration approved faster speed lines at chicken plants. Those facilities are more likely to have COVID-19 cases. *The Washington Post.* Trump administration approved faster line speeds at chicken plants - The Washington Post.

Krumel, T. P. (2017). Anti-immigration reform and reductions in welfare: Evidence from the meatpacking industry. *Choices*, *32*(1), 1–7. DOI: 10.22004/ag.econ.256579

Krumel, T. P., & Goodrich, C. (2021). *Covid-19 Working Paper: Meatpacking working conditions and the spread of COVID-19.* USDA, Economic Research Service, Covid 19 Working Paper #AP-092. COVID-19 Working Paper: Meatpacking Working Conditions and the Spread of COVID-19 (usda.gov).

Landbrugsavisen (2020, September 28). *Danish Crown kæmpede med hygiejnen under coronasmitte i Ringsted* [Danish Crown had hygiene problems during the COVID-19 outbreak in Ringsted]. Landbrugsavisen. Danish Crown kæmpede med hygiejnen under coronasmitte i Ringsted | LandbrugsAvisen.

Langhelle, O. (2002). Bærekraftig utvikling [Sustainable development]. In T. A. Benjaminsen & H. Svarstad (Eds.), *Samfunnsperspektiver på miljø og utvikling* [Societal perspectives on environment and development] (2nd ed., pp. 225–254). Universitetsforlaget.

Laughland, O., & Holpuch, A. (2020, May 2). We're modern slaves: How meat plant workers became the new frontline in Covid-19 war. *The Guardian.* 'We're modern slaves': How meat plant workers became the new frontline in Covid-19 war | Coronavirus | The Guardian.

Lussenhop, J. (2020, April 17). *Coronavirus at Smithfield pork plant: The untold story of America's biggest outbreak.* BBC News. Coronavirus at Smithfield pork plant: The untold story of America's biggest outbreak - BBC News.

Mano, A. (2020a, September 8). *Special report: How COVID-19 swept the Brazilian slaughterhouses of JBS, world's top meatpacker.* Reuters, Business News. Special Report: How COVID-19 swept the Brazilian slaughterhouses of JBS, world's top meatpacker | Reuters.

Mano, A. (2020b, November 10). *Socially conscious investors rank Brazil's JBS, BRF 'medium' risk, Minerva 'high'.* Reuters, Agriculture. Socially conscious investors rank Brazil's JBS, BRF 'medium' risk, Minerva 'high' | Reuters.

Markvardsen, C. (2020, June 22). *Tysk minister: Slagterikoncern skal betale for corona-omkostninger* [German minister says slaughterhouse must pay COVID-19 expenses]. Dr.dk. Tysk minister: Slagterikoncern skal betale for corona-omkostninger | Udland | DR.

McSweeny, E., & Young, H. (2021, September 28). 'The whole system is rotten': Life inside Europe's meat industry. *The Guardian.* 'The whole system is rotten': life inside Europe's meat industry | Meat industry | The Guardian

MercoPress (2020, July 20). *Brazilian meat plants perfect "coronavirus breeding centers", according to Labor Ministry.* MercoPress, South Atlantic News Agency. Brazilian meat plants perfect "coronavirus breeding centers", according to Labor Ministry – MercoPress.

Mota, C. V. (2020, July 22). *Covid-19 se alastra em frigoríficos e põe brasileiros e imigrantes em risco* [COVID-19 spreads in slaughterhouses and puts Brazilians and immigrants at risk]. BBC News Brasil. Covid-19 se alastra em frigoríficos e põe brasileiros e imigrantes em risco - BBC News Brasil.

Nierenberg, D. (2005). *Happier meals. Rethinking the global meat industry.* Worldwatch Paper 171. Worldwatch Institute.

Novic, Z. (2021). *Too fast, too furious: Slaughterhouse line speeds in the era of Covid-19.* [Master's thesis]. Yale School of Public Health. Too Fast, Too Furious: Slaughterhouse Line Speeds In The Era Of Covid-19 (yale.edu).

Parra, C. (2013). Social sustainability: A competing concept to social innovation? In F. Moulaert, D. MacCallum, & A. Mehmood (Eds.), *The international handbook on social innovation. Collective action, social learning and transdisciplinary research* (pp. 142–154). Edward Elgar.

Phillips, D. (2020, July 15). 'There's a direct relationship': Brazil meat plants linked to spread of COVID-19. *The Guardian.* 'There's a direct relationship': Brazil meat plants linked to spread of Covid-19 | Brazil | The Guardian.

Pina, R. (2020, June 23). *Como frigoríficos propagaram o coronavirus em pequenas cidades do pais* [How slaughterhouses spread the coronavirus in small towns across the country]. Publica. Como frigoríficos propagaram o coronavírus em pequenas cidades do país (apublica.org).

Pokora, R., Kutschbach, S., Weigl, M., Braun, D., Epple, A., Lorenz, E., Grund, S., Hecht, J., Holich, H., Rietschel, P., Schneider, F., Schmen, R., Taylor, K., & Dienstbuehl, I. (2021). Investigation of superspreading COVID-19 outbreak events in meat and poultry processing plants in Germany: A cross-sectional study. *PLoS ONE, 16*(6), 1–14. 10.1371/journal.pone.0242456

Rankin, J. (2021, October 5). EU 'failing to stop meat industry exploiting agency workers'. *The Guardian.* EU 'failing to stop meat industry exploiting agency workers' | Meat industry | The Guardian.

Redanz, M., & Rasmussen, P. (2020, August 12). *Smitteudbruddet i Ringsted: Derfor bor slagteriarbejdere i en køjeseng i årevis* [The outbreak in Ringsted: That's why slaughterhouse workers live in bunk beds for years]. Fagbladet3F. Smitteudbruddet i Ringsted: Derfor bor slagteriarbejdere i en køjeseng i årevis | Fagbladet 3F.

Redclift, M. (1987). *Sustainable development: Exploring the contradictions.* Routledge.

Reiley, L. (2020, April 28). In one month, the meat industry's supply chain broke. Here's what you need to know. *The Washington Post.* FAQ: What consumers need to know about the meat industry right now – The Washington Post.

Ritchi, H., & Roser, M. (2019). *Our world in data. Meat and dairy production.* Meat and Dairy Production – Our World in Data.

Romania Insider. (2020, April 29). *About 200 Romanian workers at slaughterhouses in Germany infected with COVID-19.* Romania Insider. About 200 Romanian workers at slaughterhouse in Germany infected with COVID-19 | Romania Insider (romania-insider.com).

Segata, J., Beck, L., & Muccillo, L. (2021). Beyond exotic wet markets: Covid-19 ecologies in the global meat-processing industry in Brazil. *eTropic, 20*(1), 94–114. 10.25120/etropic.20.1.2021.3794

Simons, J., & Lenders, D. (2020). *Covid-19 – Impact on the meat sector in Germany.* FFTC Agricultural Policy Platform (FFTC-AP). COVID-19 – Impact on the Meat Sector in Germany | FFTC Agricultural Policy Platform (FFTC-AP).

Solomon, E., Hopkins, V., & Vladkov, A. (2021, January 8). Inside Germany's abattoirs: The human cost of cheap meat. *Financial Times Magazine*. Inside Germany's abattoirs: the human cost of cheap meat | Financial Times (ft.com).

Staunton, B. (2021). Change a long time coming for subcontracted slaughterhouse workers. *HesaMag*, *23*, 14–17. HM23_Change a long time coming for subcontracted slaughterhouse workers_2021_0.pdf (etui.org).

Steinfeld, H., Gerber, P., Wassenaar, T., Castel, W., Rosales, M., & de Haan, C. (2006). *Livestock's long shadow. Environmental issues and options*. FAO. Livestock's long shadow: environmental issues and options (fao.org).

Taylor, C. A., Boulos, C., & Almond, D. (2020). Livestock plants and COVID-19 transmission. *PNAS*, *117*(50), 31706–31715. 10.1073/pnas.2010115117

Telford, T., Kindy, K., & Bogage, J. (2020, April 29). Trump orders meat plants to stay open in pandemic. *The Washington Post*. Trump orders meat plants to say open, citing Defense Production Act – The Washington Post.

Tiirikainen, M., & Koch, K. (2020, August 8). *Derfor lukker Danish Crown i Ringsted – coronasmitte begyndte at springe* [Why Danish Crown in Ringsted is closing: COVID-19 infections started to jump]. TV2 Øst. Derfor lukker Danish Crown i Ringsted – coronasmitte begyndte at springe | TV2 ØST (tv2east.dk).

US Congress. (2021, October 27). *Memorandum*. Congress of the United States, House of Representatives, Select Committee on the Coronavirus Crisis. 2021.10.27 Meatpacking Report.Final_.pdf (house.gov).

Wagner, B., & Hassel, A. (2016). Posting, subcontracting and low-wage employment in the German meat industry. *Transfer: European Review of Labour and Research*, *22*(2), 163–178. 10.1177%2F1024258916636012

Wagner, I., & Refslund, B. (2016). Understanding the diverging trajectories of slaughterhouse work in Denmark and Germany: A power resource approach. *European Journal of Industrial Relations*, 22(4), 335–351. 10.1177%2F0959680116682109

Waltenburg, M. A., Victoroff, T., Rose, C. E., et al. (2020). *Update: COVID-19 among workers in meat and poultry processing facilities – United States, April-May 2020*. Morbidity and Mortality Weekly Report. Center for Disease Control and Prevention. Update: COVID-19 Among Workers in Meat and Poultry Processing Facilities – United States, April–May 2020 | MMWR (cdc.gov).

Weis, T. (2014). *The ecological hoofprint: The global burden of industrial livestock*. Zed Books.

Whittail, M., & Trinczek, R. (2020). Structural characteristics and industrial relations in the pork value chain: The case of Germany. In P. Campanella & D. Dazzi (Eds.), *Meat-up Ffire. Fairness, freedom and industrial relations across Europe: Up and down the meat value chain* (pp. 103–137). FrancoAngeli.

World Commission on Environment and Development. (1987). *Our common future*. Oxford University Press.

11 The COVID-19 lockdown and pathways for sustainable transition

Jesper Holm

Introduction

When responses to the COVID-19 pandemic during the years 2020 and 2021 began in earnest, with an effective lockdown[1] and state of emergency policies, a striking number of personally articulated comments on adapting to the situation and expectations of great changes grew among otherwise pessimistic voices in the very depths of the despair. The expectation was that public policies could, in fact, rapidly develop new capabilities to break with long-term, systemic lock-ins, especially a break for stronger climate change mitigation. For decades, path dependency in societal practices from commuting to housing and energy consumption has threatened planetary boundaries, local and socio-psychological resilience and public health. Presently, in 2022–2023, the pandemic period is still referred to as a game changer for the acceleration of new modes of living on Earth (Latour & Schultz, 2022), and the governing politics of, for example, climate change mitigation (European Union [EU], 2022). In the European Union, a *New Green Deal* for all business sectors is still being enacted in its sub-programmes as a post-COVID kick-start investment push, involving, e.g., circular economy and enhanced biodiversity, areas that are normally not connected to economic growth. The European Union, United States and Western welfare states seem to have discovered and shown during pandemic times that budgeting for far-reaching plans in policies, such as the New Green Deal in the European Union, is in fact possible. As Hartmut Rosa (2020, p. 2) put it, 'With the advent of coronavirus, we all of a sudden see that within a few weeks, political action can regain supremacy and gain control over activities in all spheres.'

The role of hope for game-changing in hitherto path-dependent health and environment regimes is highly interesting in times of despair such as the COVID-19 period. What is the basis for this kind of hope in terms of sustainable transition during and following COVID-19? How can research contribute to the understanding of the role of these enthusiastic calls for deep change?

This chapter contributes to section three of the book by exploring the anticipation of sustainability-oriented alterations of politics and everyday

DOI: 10.4324/9781003441915-14

life, during and after the lockdown period of 2020–2022. What are the places, positions, and discourses of these expectations, and which pandemic factors fostered them? This chapter aims to reflect on the possible importance and prospects of broadly mobilised hope and its background in the study of transition. It may lead to a more general question: Does a severe, embodied social and health crisis generate different game-changing dynamics than an economic crisis, as often claimed? Could the COVID-19 lockdown result in new types of inputs to the theoretical understanding of the preconditions for radical change?

Here, the focus on the theme of the book 'COVID-19, welfare and health' is related to sustainable transition that, in many aspects, incorporates environmental health as '... an interdisciplinary academic field, an area of research, and an area of applied public health practice' (Frumkin, 2005, p. xxxi). Environmental health covers structures and practices that influence the parts of the environment important to our health and well-being, be it urban structures, chemicals in the ocean, traffic, work, climate, air and water pollution, or contaminants in our food. In 2016, the growing attention to environmental health merged the Shanghai Declaration on Health Promotion into the 2030 Agenda for Sustainable Development (World Health Organization [WHO], 2016). Health promotion methods and strategies have thus become part of the actions required to achieve the 17 Sustainable Development Goals (SDG17) (United Nations [UN], 2015).

The chapter takes a cross-disciplinary approach across health promotion and social science to analyse the issue in four different steps:

1 The background summarises the overall problem focus of sustainable transition, then introduces two schools of thought that align well among theories of radical societal change: sustainable transition theory (e.g. Geels, Kemp, and Grin) and critical state theory (e.g. Jessop, Meadowcraft, Eckersley, and Jänicke). These theories are interdisciplinary and systems-oriented, analysing a variety of circumstances at a location in order to generate sustainable transition on different scales of society. They deal with the kinds of social circumstances, politics/state, and socio-technical conditions that may uphold a transformative period. They also delve into the kinds of dynamics in the triangle of civic society-market-state that open windows of opportunity to move towards radical changes.
2 Then follows an analysis of the media-covered personal sense of resilience and openings for radical change to happen during the lockdown period. Document studies then follow new political claims and programmes for a radical shift in policy interventions, echoing parts of COVID-19 policies. Here, empirical findings on restarting society through EU or national state interventionism point to signs of radical policy interventions during the pandemic and post-lockdown.
3 The next section discusses a shift in observation that perceives discourses of civic and institutional claims as voices of hope for transitions to come,

their focus and circumstances leading to a semi-philosophical reflection on the deep importance of hope to spur innovations in times of crisis and to provide cheer to cognitive desolation.
4 Finally, the conclusion elaborates on the findings of the potentiality of hope.

Background: Theories of radical change

The call for radical change

Politics for a radical shift in societal dynamics towards strong sustainability have in recent years led marginal deep ecologists and like-minded groups to become a common point of focus in addition to numerous scientific evaluations, official environmental status reports, and policy documents on how poorly states and international regimes have managed to tackle the climate and biodiversity crises along with related environmental health problems. Today, the magnitude of climate change and other global issues is perceived to exacerbate the planet's inability to sustain humanity in its current version, as evidenced by the EU Biodiversity Strategy 2030 (EU, 2022) or the latest International Panel on Climate Change (IPCC) report. In the latter, path dependency, narrow sector focus, and poorly developed management capacity are criticised (IPCC, 2022) for having contributed to the disastrous global resource, biodiversity, and climate problems. Scientists such as Koch (2020); O'Neill (2015), and Pichler et al. (2017) have more deeply exposed the problems of policy responses to date, exploring the invalidity of the notion of ecological modernisation,[2] i.e. a belief system of gradual decoupling between economic growth and material input. Perhaps more authoritative is the Human Development Report from the United Nations Development Programme (UNDP, 2020), which for the first time compiled global data on the link between social and economic development on the one hand and ecological impact on the other. These data indicate that there are currently no examples of states where there are well-developed social rights and healthy economic development combined with a low ecological footprint. In other words, green growth and ecological modernisation have not yet been successful.

To bring their environmental performances, especially their matter and energy throughputs, in line with ecological thresholds, and to reach United Nations climate targets (IPCC, 2022), rich countries would need to degrow (Koch, 2020).

> Climate change has caused substantial damages, and increasingly irreversible losses, in terrestrial, freshwater and coastal and open ocean marine ecosystems ... The extent and magnitude of climate change impacts are larger than estimated in previous assessments ... Widespread deterioration of ecosystem structure and function, resilience and natural adaptive capacity, as

> well as shifts in seasonal timing have occurred due to climate change … with adverse socioeconomic consequences … Actions that focus on sectors and risks in isolation and on short-term gains often lead to maladaptation if long-term impacts of the adaptation option and long-term adaptation commitment are not taken into account … .
>
> (IPCC, 2022, pp. 4–6)

The Stockholm Resilience Centre has provided much of the background to the currently most-used scientific insights in terms of the limits to the growth of global earth systems, dubbed the planetary boundaries (Steffen et al., 2015). Such credible sources give strong signals about the global limits to material growth. However, there is no consensus. Yet the notion of limits is today more widely popular than in the 1970s when the Club of Rome launched their book *Limits to Growth* (Meadows et al., 1972). I build here upon these partly normative assumptions of a necessary, fixed, material growth framework for each nation today, this gives us a picture of the nearly utopian magnitude of interventions and change that will have to take place. However, parts of critical state theory and transition theory can guide us to the preconditions for a sustainable transition.

State theory

In general, social science theorists have explored critical insights into state failure or implementation deficits within state theory (see Blühdorn, 2007; Jänicke, 1990). However, here we focus on options for greening the state to redirect society and analytical attempts over the last three decades in critical state theory.

The Danish social scientist Jesper Pedersen (1991) was one of the first to outline ideas for a cooperative ecological state capable of handling ecological crises, a state with several instances of negotiating checks and balances for distributing environmental goods and resources. Similar ideas came from a group organised under the European Union's Fifth Environmental Research Programme on the Ecological State in 1995–1997, where nature's sinks, biodiversity, and sustainable resource handling were to be the founding principles of multi-level governance. The Australian political scientist John Dryzek (1997) proposed a mix of discourses on *green rationalism* and *survivalism* that a *green state* might successfully follow. Here, the insights focus on political ecology and power structures behind the capture of the environmental agenda by the market economy and the political room for manoeuvre, given absolute material limits.

Barry and Eckersly (2005) gathered state analysts to support a theory of the *environmental state* to demolish ecological modernisation[iii] and enhance political room for manoeuvre among green forces of change. Their arguments see the potential of altered politics during the age of economic crisis, through political forces opposing corporate power to downgrade neoliberal politics in environmental health issues. Additionally, social movements, socio-economic forces, and alternative strategically oriented formations of central actors need to adopt a stronger role in politics, which are all elements that borrow their thinking from the neo-Gramscian philosophy of politics and state (D'Alisa & Kallis, 2020; Jessop, 2008). In 2016 and 2020, the journal *Environmental Politics* published two themed issues, where the development of a new form of state outside the growth society made its appearance with transition-theoretical angles on politics in sustainable transition, as well as counter-growth-based ideological-political measures. Similarly, a large number of relevant articles about the state and counter-growth have been published in the journal *Ecological Economics* since 2020. In Denmark, a book on the sustainable state (Willig & Blok, 2020) and a special issue of *Samfundsøkonomen* (2022) discuss the role of a new state in sustainable transition.

Most literature focuses on greening or sustaining the state. A new state's functioning would enable it to tackle the types of crises mentioned above. It would manage to redistribute economic resources to protect biosystems, citizens and natural resources, dematerialise growth, and install policies for the good life and sustainable households. This is typical in state theories initiated by strategic manoeuvring from counter-growth forces and public deliberation and installing various types of deliberative democracy. Important outcomes for citizens include support for non-consumption-based life policies, culture, shorter working hours, a radical redistribution policy, cooperatives to run production, and state takeover of key industries (D'Alisa & Kallis, 2020; Koch, 2020). Only a few studies elaborate on how to design the institutional configuration of the state itself (Holm, 2022). Accordingly, state theory provides a positive vision of new missions to be accomplished and gives priority to democratic bottom-up forces that may generate this transition. Nevertheless, we find no insight into what kind of opening or situation will motivate, engage, and galvanise forces and citizens to enable a green state to emerge.

Transition theory

Another way to conceive radical change towards a more sustainable society follows more specific changes to socio-technical practices in various areas from everyday life to energy supply systems. The success of transition theory and sustainable transition studies, since they were initiated in the late 1990s by Dutch (e.g. Geels, 2004) and Belgian scholars (e.g. Kemp et al., 1998), is their intriguing focus on concrete everyday life and production activities and on market dynamics and technological innovations among small frontrunner companies and their networks, eventually influencing the predominant regimes of various sectors such as farming and transport. The role of the state may take many forms but is more discreet than in state theory. Transition studies are now part of the EU analytical and strategic vocabulary, probably because of their neutral capability to provide various real-time socio-technical tracks of the study of systems such as commuting, clothing, and housing in liberal market systems. There is different advice on the path that a liberal state in a market system could follow in transition policies and network-driven management of the market towards more sustainable socio-technical niches or regimes around sectors, consumption areas, and industries (Geels, 2004; Geels & Kemp, 2012; Holm et al., 2014). Numerous studies have addressed the preconditions for the emergence of more sustainable transition processes and how an environmental state, typically in partnership with companies, science and civic groups, may deliberately conduct such processes over a series of steps (Kemp & Rotmans, 2001; Köhler et al., 2019; Voß & Kemp, 2006). Scholars of transition have provided a multi-level model, where regime shift processes, such as establishing a low-waste economy, organic food farming, and non-chemical systems, depend on a dynamic interplay between socio-technical regimes and socio-political landscapes and niches (Geels, 2004; Kemp & Rotmans, 2001).

To give a case example, current socio-technical systems of the health sector can be characterised by a dominant regime of hospitalisation and medicalisation, sustained and supported by predominant medical actors, institutions and regulations (Broerse & Grin, 2017). This regime is maintaining the technological trajectories, e.g., the birth-giving regime, standardised medication methods for wicked health problems, or Fordist IT platforms handling bodies of diseases (patients). The dominant regime may change through innovative processes performed by networks of the actors involved in different dimensions of the regime, e.g. industry, policy, science, or client culture. These processes may, however, suddenly be influenced by changes in the landscape such as the COVID-19 lockdown, creating new conditions for development and offering windows of opportunity for new health and disease handling technology systems. Regime changes can stem from niches of emerging technologies/practices, which may be included in a transformation of the regime or may put the regime under pressure by offering an alternative. Processes of niche creation, learning processes, translation, and transfer of ideas are very important for the transition, and innovative actors within and outside the dominant regime are of interest here (Geels, 2004; Kemp et al., 2007). Niches in health systems often develop from research and development experimentation among social entrepreneurs. Local projects and initiatives may serve the function of socio-technical experimentations, where combinations of new technologies and living practices unfold and develop into alternative options. They can be described as situated transition places established as specific configurations (Holm et al., 2014), in which health communities, user-driven eco-settlements, institutional funds that interact with municipalities, and specific parts of the food, nutrition, and health industries define contextualised socio-technical experiments (Brown & Vergragt, 2008). In this way, they form sites of situated learning.

Transition theory gives promising inputs to understand the development of new trajectories in socio-technical practices that in time may deliver more sustainable energy, housing, and mobility paths. However, it does not deal with degrowth, but favours actors engaged with technology, manufacturing, services, or farming, and tends to build on a very rationalistic approach to motivation (Gram-Hannsen, 2014).

Analysis: Signs of radical changes

Signs of change in everyday life

> In Paris, they can hear the birds singing. The Italians sing from the balconies. Children are with their parents. Many more have time to enjoy the Danish spring, bake muffins, cook together and play board games. Garden owners can start doing the spring work. The world has become slower and closer. In the midst of the COVID-19 crisis, we can also experience normally suppressed things and linering in our hectic demanding everyday life. Moreover, not least, we see thousands volunteering for emergency preparedness and neighbourhood help groups. The care and empathy extend beyond those closest to you.
>
> (Belling, 2020)

The changes in daily life during COVID-19, for most Danes, were of a sensory, experiential kind, of which several dimensions were celebrated as character-transforming. We discuss selected signs of radical change that for some represent the dark side of the pandemic, while for others they display a bright side. Working from home and being out of work have been celebrated as creating images of a different kind of family life, more time with friends and family, and a decrease in work-life imbalances. On the other hand, there was the invasion of privacy from a job and school perspective, stress for parents, and deprivation of young people for different reasons (Clemensen et al., 2021). Thus, the focus is on claimed 'goods', despite all the 'bads'. Deep problematic socio-economic and health impacts emerged from the same changes, unevenly distributed among social groups.[3] The shutdown of commuting, jobs, schools, flights, and entertainment combined with radical self-isolation led to wide-ranging alterations, all resulting from the emergency COVID-19 policies of the Danish state (Petersen & Roepstorf, 2020). Working from home has been shown to continue after the pandemic, with a doubling of numbers on average from 2019 to late 2021 (from 100 000 to 200 000 out of 2.8 million jobs in Denmark). Personal benefits include a better work-life balance, enhanced freedom in jobs, and relief from the stress of commuting. In the wake of COVID-19, many companies and government organisations have taken new decisions about what the physical workplace should look like and be able to provide in the future, and the best extent of working from home. In addition, in many places a new design model for workplace and home has emerged, where the company is mainly a meeting place and the home serves as the location for individual work. In shutdown periods, 680 000 to 830 000 people worked at home on a normal working day, thus enabling a new culture to mature (Dansk Industri, 2021). Although there is much discussion of whether the continued work-from-home culture is problematic or not for the working environment and health, COVID-19 was a game changer for popular wishes to lower working hours, at a time when the government wanted to increase working hours for Danes.

Some research projects unfolded the importance of COVID-19 for changes in political attitudes and on public media debates on linkages between the pandemic and climate crisis, where especially one study is of interest here. Toft and Nielsen (2023) did a thorough study of media coverage that gave new insights to the importance of a disaster's impact on narratives on relations between COVID-19, biodiversity loss, nature exploration, and political hubris. For citizens, the pandemic seems to have raised the number of citizens that aims for post-COVID-19 more slow living, fewer travelling, and politically a higher number favour greener tax politics, improved space for nature, and aim for a green re-start after COVID-19 (ibid, pp. 12–15).

The withdrawal of all giant cruise ships (463 in 2017) that used to be in Port Copenhagen's three cruise ship terminals, as well as in Aarhus and Aalborg, was a dramatic change. The often-criticised tourism in different inner-city areas of Copenhagen and Aarhus suddenly vanished as the ships stopped bringing large groups of guided tourists who took up noticeable urban space. Instead, urban space became available for locals and guests from other parts of Denmark in the staycation period of COVID-19. The bonus positive impact of lower air pollution from small particles, sulphur dioxide, and nitrogen oxides (NOx) from bunker-oil-fuelled ship motors running around the clock was celebrated as growing public, political, and scientific attention to the non-regulated pollution from the tourism sector emerged (Cherét, 2020). Total emissions from cruise ships in Copenhagen Port in 2017 were 284.5 tons of NOx and 10.0 tons of PM2.5. By way of comparison, total emissions from all sources within the large calculation grid in Copenhagen were 1669 tons of NOx and 175 tons of PM2.5 (Jensen et al., 2019). The greatly reduced leisure and travel activity also highlighted the massive socio-economic importance of tourism and exposed its negative climate and environmental footprints, which had been neglected in Denmark for decades (Holm & Kaae, 2017).

Another very visible radical change was the streets that were periodically almost empty of cars, which encouraged more cycling and walking in urban areas. For people commuting by car, there was less traffic. Overall, bicycle traffic increased by almost 10% from 2019 to 2020, and pedestrian traffic by almost 50% as an annual average (Nielsen & Christiansen, 2021). Calculated only for the shutdown periods, pedestrian, and bicycle traffic more than doubled in many places. The reason was primarily an increase in leisure/exercise trips, but the bike also took market share from public transport, especially after the introduction of the mask requirement in August 2020. Clear blue sky, birdsong audible in cities across long distances, and increased outdoor activities in nature among Danes became the common celebration of pandemic culture (Friluftsrådet, 2023; Naturstyrelsen, 2020), and this has been maintained but on a lower level in post-pandemic times (Naturstyrelsen, 2022). Staycation, a new phenomenon among the many travelling Danes of staying home instead of travelling abroad, was also a result of banning foreign travel during COVID-19. Usually, 45% of Danes travel abroad for their holidays, but this dropped to 10% during the pandemic. However, the staycation culture is expected to fade away in 2023 (Dansk Erhverv, 2022). The most tangible environmental benefit from the COVID-19 lockdown has been the reduction in air pollution in Denmark compared to previous years, and for the first time, it measured below the EU ambient air quality standards for most substances (Ellermann et al., 2022).

As for everyday life at home, indoor living has come into focus during the various shutdowns regarding space for homeworking for all family members. Outdoor living has also taken on new dimensions in relation to contact at a distance and recreational opportunities without the risk of infection. Therefore, experiences from the lockdown and spatial distancing norms have already influenced urban planning and housing patterns with more attention to providing space in housing (Bygherreforeningen, 2021). There is a new trend whereby architecture and planning of housing are not only valued for the quality of the individual building but also in relation to opportunities for community-building between the inhabitants, urban cohesion (Mossin et al., 2022), and access to practical involvement with nature and gardening). COVID-19 has led to this trend because the whole of Denmark experienced indoor isolation with limited options for social interaction and outdoor activities. Moreover, the pandemic has proved to be a game changer by fostering this move away from a hitherto compartmentalised individualistic focus in construction policies.

Signs of change in politics

Diverse Danish environmental NGOs (such as the Klima- og Omstillingsrådet [Climate and Transition Council], NOAH [Friends of the Earth], Omstilling Nu! [Transition Now!], and the green think tank CONCITO), business organisations (such as Dansk Energi [Danish Energy]), and researchers (Pedersen, 2020; Willig & Blok, 2020) have raised their voices for learning from the effective altered health policies during COVID-19 to achieve a sustainable transition perspective. The NGO Climate and Transition Council states:

> Social and traditional media quickly spread stories about citizens who valued aspects of life during the suspension, with associated new work patterns, habits, communities and consumption patterns. In addition,

> researchers, political elites and civil society have pointed out that the COVID-19 crisis should be seen as an opportunity to change our society in a desirable direction with slogans such as 'green restart' and 'build back better'.
>
> (Schultz et al., 2020)

The European Environment Agency (EEA) and the European Commission have also expressed ideas for a green restart of society post-COVID-19 in the direction of policies for transition in biodiversity and the climate crisis, work-life balancing, new green jobs, and higher SDG17 target achievement. With disillusionment of the otherwise normal politics of necessity, new openings for green politics of transition have emerged. According to interviews with Danish professors Ove Kaj Pedersen (Pedersen, 2020) and Mikkel Vedby Rasmussen (Jacobsen, 2021), policies and plans can make a difference. In an open call with the press on 6 February 2021, more than 700 researchers pointed out the government's capacity for action during COVID-19 and how it could be transferred to the climate crisis. As Professor Bruno Latour put it,

> The first lesson the coronavirus has taught us is also the most astounding: we have actually proven that it is possible, in a few weeks, to put an economic system on hold everywhere in the world and at the same time, a system that we were told, it was impossible to slow down or redirect. … If in a month or two, millions of humans are capable of learning how to social distance at the blow of a whistle, to space themselves for greater solidarity, to stay home so as not to overload the hospitals, then it is easy to imagine the power of transformation that these new protective measures have against bringing back business as usual.
>
> (Latour, 2020)

Radical aspirations for change can be found in the European Union's post-COVID-19 policy documents such as the sustainable food strategy *From Farm to Fork* from 2020, part of the *NextGenerationEU* recovery fund (EU, 2022). The fund aims to support the EU member states in a green kick-start, also known as the *New Green Deal* regime. Again, we find ideologies of strategic leapfrogging infused with great expectations.

> NextGenerationEU is more than a recovery plan – it is a once in a lifetime chance to emerge stronger from the pandemic, transform our economies and societies, and design a Europe that works for everyone. We have everything we need to make this happen. We have a vision; we have a plan and we have agreed to invest €806.9 billion together.
>
> (EU, 2022, front page of website)

The EEA highlights these initiatives from the pandemic experience:

> EU Member States have willingly taken measures against COVID-19 that have had enormous economic costs, along with creating the risk of economic recession and severe unemployment. Can a similar level of responsiveness be mobilised for achieving transitions to sustainability ... ? The World Health Organization estimate of seven million annual deaths due to air pollution would also justify strict measures.
>
> (European Environmental Agency (EEA), 2021, p. 4)

In leading articles in *Nature* and *Science* from 2020 to 2022, some calls for optional green policy measures started taking shape with the zoonotic background of COVID-19. There is no general consensus about the causal origins of the virus, but consensus does exist that it is of animal origin and crossed species boundaries to infect humans, either before or after it evolved to its current pathogenic state. Viruses can very rapidly spread in a globalised economic system with high levels of interconnectedness and mobility (Keesing & Ostfeld, 2021). A key question over the past decade has been whether the decline in biodiversity increases the pool of pathogens that can be transmitted from animals to humans. 'There is increasing evidence that global environmental change, the loss of biodiversity and its associated regulatory services, and the emergence, or increase in the prevalence of zoonotic diseases are linked' (Lawler et al., 2021, p. 9). Work by Jones and colleagues suggests that a loss in biodiversity usually results in a few species replacing many, and these species tend to be the ones hosting pathogens that can spread to humans (Jones et al., 2008). Addressing zoonotic causes of human health has led to calls for change in strategies such as addressing the concept of 'One Health', which recognises the interconnection between people, animals, plants, and their shared environment, with the goal to achieve optimal health outcomes (Bonilla-Aldana et al., 2020).

In the journal *International Health Promotion* from 2020 and 2021, viewpoints on learning from COVID-19 build on health promotion discourses: there is a call for a re-orientation of the current healthcare system towards better connection to local communities and citizens' ability to manage their health themselves during a pandemic (Van den Broucke, 2020). In healthcare professions, discussions focus on the need to uphold the principles of the Ottawa Charter, reflected in the countries' reactions to COVID-19; several authors see a showdown with the long-term paradigmatic commitment to the individual citizen in health care (e.g. Cardona, 2020)

To sum up, we have witnessed various types of experiences in our daily lives, such as substantial sensory changes for the betterment of our environment and well-being, and we have heard a choir of green believers with declarations and demands from all parts of the policy matrix for robust governance for sustainable transition and the alteration of behaviouristic approaches.

Radical changes perceived as hope

In several studies of disasters and their policy implications 'disasters function as prisms that allow us to see how tacit structures and taken-for-granted processes of organising, planning and dealing with societal questions are in fact harmful [...] Sudden expressions of underlying (failing) structures and processes characterising the societies in which they occur.' (Toft & Nielsen, 2023 p. 4). What is new is a mix of jointly experienced, stated, and politically proclaimed windows for a greener and more resilient future. COVID-19 has shown us experiences of other conceivable development paths, and that real planning is objectively possible. The extent to which we seem to have changed our image of us-in-society during the lockdown is noticeable. Our radius of physical movement, the purpose of our movement, ordinary social gatherings, the living space of couples, patterns of leaving the home, and the roles of parents and children have changed markedly and are explicitly linked to societal considerations. Maybe in times of other catch-all crises such as the Ukrainian war, a similar urgent call for a response is heard, such as demands for radical policies for the acceleration of renewable energy. In Denmark, we disagree on whether we should call the actions during COVID-19 intensified governmentalisation, a state-led shutdown of democracy and freedom, a deep state, or an exercise of responsible authority. The result was that performance speed slowed down, racing between home and work decreased, hours in traffic jams disappeared, and demands for omnipotent self-realisation were removed – for a while. Firstly, this means that from the highest health authority to calls from the retail trade for self-governance, we received a series of communications to rethink and extend our consideration in normal body-distance-social interaction to the invisible other and to the weak in society. Secondly, it means a short-lived and sudden (but not for all) deceleration of imbalances in working life (Rosa, 2020), and a form of societal contemplation with simpler lifestyles as a result. It is this opening of another opportunity for existence, a movement sideways through the social order, and a move away from the status quo in times of urgency, which may have fostered an affective reaction such as hope. Thus, hope as a starting point for political and everyday motivation, mobilisation, and reflection on the possible paths of the promoted changes necessary for sustainable transition needs to be studied more deeply.

The British sociologist/political scientist Bob Jessop would call the above-mentioned issues signs of focused, hope-based ideal-type thinking, or normative-cognitive mental notions that both seek to summarise existing developments and anticipate desired potential tracks of development (Jessop, 2012). Such imaginaries are not uniform but can accommodate a number of variations within the regime of political transition strategies, in line with Dryzeck's discursive patterns (1997) and Oomen and colleagues' (2022) powerful analysis of how imagined futures become socially performative. They bring together a few phenomena, and discourses in a heterogeneous regime that encourages surveys and systematic studies of areas of society and thus interventions.

> Imaginaries often include prospective as well as descriptive elements, anticipating or recommending new lines of action, that may guide present and future (non-) decisions and (in)actions in a world pregnant with possibilities. ... Crises tend to create profound cognitive, strategic, and practical disorientation by disrupting actors' sedimented views of the world, including their various social imaginaries. They disturb prevailing meta-narratives, theoretical frameworks, policy paradigms, and/or everyday life and create space for proliferation (variation) in crisis interpretations, drawing on different imaginaries, only some of which get selected as the basis for 'imagined recoveries' to be translated into economic strategies and policies.
>
> (Jessop, 2012, p. 3)

Radical social imaginaries have for decades echoed among enclaves or social movements but have never been seriously articulated or regularly heard outside deep ecologists' communication to a wider sustainability-oriented public. Since the 1970s, real-utopian dreams of green change have lost attention (see Engholm, 2023; Holm & Kristensen, 2014; Martell, 2018). Generally, only very small groups of privileged ecologists or bohemians articulate short periodic hopes of realising radical changes in our way of life, whether in terms of increased equality, sustainable consumption/production, or strengthened health resilience. It is very rare for these enclaves to momentarily link with broad groups or institutions, in order to mobilise political discussion on sustainable transition efforts. However, ordinary people frequently engage in utopian hope and thinking, and utopian hope may thus be an important affective driver of social change. As imagined possible worlds, 'real-utopias' may motivate individuals' engagement with society in much the same way as possible selves can play a significant role in individuals' lives (Fernando et al., 2014; Wright, 2010).

The principle of hope was formulated philosophically and ethically as a particular interdisciplinary way of thinking by the German philosopher Ernst Bloch in the 1950s, based on history, anthropology, politics, and religiosity (Bloch, 1970). In his opinion, the 'objectively real possible' is long-term hope. For example, we can observe it during the current climate change and the pandemic crisis, through the same lens. The framework and conditions that previously seemed unshakeable are now proving changeable.

> According to Bloch, hope as a principle is present in every action as a driving force and structure. The principle of hope anchors a fundamental observation of our lives, our world and our whole being as being unfinished, in constant motion. With this, hope is an ever-present crack in reality. Hope is what shows a way out. It points to something different

> that is not yet present but may already be felt and recognized as a deficiency in the current situation. [...] The time of hope thus appears as a complex, contradictory now, [...] The time of hope [is] a presence that is never finished and closed, but always emerging to something else, in the process of realizing new hopes and in combating new causes of the opposites to hope, fear.
>
> (Nygaard, 2014, p. 12)

Articulation of ideological hope in political discourses has also been nurtured in periods of visionary, political declamations such as the *Brundtland Report on Sustainable Development* or the *Ottawa Charter for Health Promotion*, both from the United Nations in 1986. They build on the same holistic policy narrative and regime of visionary development notions instead of the hitherto risk-reduction politics of reducing 'bads' (Almlund & Holm, 2015; Holm et al., 2015). Currently, some policy acclamations of hope around the UN's 17 sustainability goals (UN, 2015) and the 2015 Paris Agreement on climate change remain, hope that the governments of the world community would now finally deliver what was promised in the Kyoto Protocol and Agenda 21 in 1992 (Ministry of Climate, Energy and Supply, 2021). Blühdorn and many others would call this an eternal simulation of sustainability politics (Blühdorn, 2007). Unsurprisingly, only a few of the hopes and ideas from the 17 sustainable development goals and the Paris agreement have been converted into convincing, substantial policies in Denmark or in the EU, under what Dryzek (1997) called the dominance of pragmatism.

Considering everything discussed above, the COVID-19 pandemic has also generated hope among a broader audience for deeper systemic changes, which comes on top of even formal political confrontations with our basic societal practices and regulatory institutions, such as the 2022 IPCC policy recommendations (IPCC, 2022) or EU's biodiversity and circular economy programmes. A growing consensus in Denmark has started to confront the Ministry of Finance's growth models in the Danish Parliament, the throw-away culture in general, or the displacement of nature by industrial agriculture and urbanisation. It is this very broadly articulated hope that has become a starting point to investigate new pathways for sustainable transition, firstly in the everyday sense of another way of life being possible, secondly in policy statements, and finally in real politics. However, the deep radical transition towards sustainable pathways has not yet occurred.

Conclusion

The deeper the crisis (e.g. climate and biodiversity) is rooted in the system, the more profound and radical are the demands for change, but the harder it is to see any realisation of realistic systemic change. When a sudden meltdown in realities evolves all over society, such as the COVID-19 lockdown, potential relief may come as envisaged windows of a possible other world, but only if human disasters are on hold. This affective reaction combined with great expectations from policy changes may generate hope, exclaimed at the same time as despair and fear following the horrifying rise in illness and long-term health impacts and deaths from COVID-19 – but in other places. This result resembles the findings from Toft and Nielsen (2023) from a policy choice view, on the role of disasters in creating options:

> [… .] how focusing events can have second-order effects on other policy areas by revealing root causes of the focusing event itself. It thereby contributes to the multiple stream approach within agenda-setting theory to understanding the nexus of disasters and policy by refining the concept of focusing events.

The emergence of a collective form of hope in times of deep crisis such as the lockdown seems to be generated from the presence of a multi-layered break with path dependency. On the individual level, this was manifested in more comfortable routines, sensing, socialising, and work-life rhythms, which also related to a spatial, environmental level: cleaner air, car-free streets, social distance, or the more strongly sensed presence of nature in one's environment. On the institutional policy level, this was seen as new far-reaching plans, policies and visioning, which broke with the previous politics of economic 'necessities'. Hope was thus not only present at the individual level but also at the institutional level. In the sociology of expectations, this could mean wishful enactments of a desired future that generates legitimation and attracts interest, or the imaginative power we see in visions like sociotechnical imaginaries (Jasanoff & Kim, 2009) and imagined futures. Hope during the pandemic crisis embodied affective experiences of resilience, as normal politics deteriorated, and real politics came closer to mirroring the language of deep transition in real-utopian dimensions (Wright, 2010).

The COVID-19 crisis and lockdown may, for the parts of the population outside hospitals and key industrial sectors, in this perspective have resembled Hartmut Rosa's notion of resonance – stormy and destructive, but at the same time providing space and options for an improved personal outreach, embedded in our social environment. This collective hope based upon a sudden opening for entwining again with the Earth (Latour) seems like an overlooked initiating, potentially empowering, motor that may support a game change towards individually, socially and politically motivated engagement in realising sustainable transition. Oomen et al. (2022) takes us deep into theories of hope and staging agency around various dramaturgical regimes, enabling possibilities for action. However, here we see a non-intentional identification; the creation and dissemination of alternative images of the future becomes stronger when these images resemble a suddenly altered current. In this way, a new form of space for action may evolve to address our deliberations and projected possibilities, thus enacting an envisaged future in the present (Oomen et al., 2022).

Approaches from state theory and transition theory provide alternative paths by which sustainable states and arenas for socio-technical change could set a new course towards sustainable transition, as an alternative to the magnitude of the various current crises. Considering the repeated returns to ecological modernisation pathways of business-as-usual, the overwhelming challenges seem enormous and unaffordable. To some degree, we saw the barriers suddenly washed away during the COVID-19 lockdown. Therefore, for a while this fostered substantive hopes as affective and political reactions. As shown, the two theories of radical change do not dwell on such a philosophical issue as the role of hope during game-changing events on a societal scale. Research would benefit from further studies of grand narratives or imagined futures of structural change, and whether they are reflected in everyday aspirations for resilience, when sudden radical changes take place.

Notes

1 In Denmark, the public response to warnings was comparatively strong and effective, especially in the initial quarantine periods, which effectively contained the spread of the disease, followed by a high vaccination rate (see the contribution from Sørensen and Thualagant). In addition, even when the scale of the disease reached pandemic level, a significant number of people did (and continue to) strictly follow the recommendations.

2 A belief system of global, green eternal growth is an option if science and technology is politically allowed to have full influence on development

3 From hermeneutics, we know about the problem of bias in our observations. The same holds true for research. This is of great importance as what I learnt from the COVID-19 pandemic is linked to my own position as a full-time professor during lockdown with a favourable housing situation in the countryside.

References

Almlund, P., & Holm J. (2015). Post Rio and Ottawa policy – Communication for deliberation. *Journal of Transdisciplinary Environmental Studies*, *15*(2), 19–35.

Barry, J., & Eckersley, R. (eds.) (2005). The State and the Global Ecological Crisis. The MIT Press.

Belling, L. (2020, June 12). *Kan Corona lære os noget om håndtering af klimakrisen?* [Can COVID-19 teach us something about dealing with the climate crisis?] A blogger's note. https://fremtidenivorehaender.dk/corona-klimakrisen/

Bloch, E. (1970). *The principle of hope*. Cambridge University Press.

Blühdorn, I. (2007). Sustaining the unsustainable: Symbolic politics and the politics of simulation. *Environmental Politics*, *16*(2), 251–275.

Bonilla-Aldana, D. K., Dhama, K., & Rodriguez-Morales, A. J. (2020). Revisiting the one health approach in the context of COVID-19: A look into the ecology of this emerging disease. *Advances in Animal and Veterinary Sciences*, *8*(3), 234–237.

Broerse, J. E. W., & Grin, J. (Eds.). (2017). *Toward sustainable transitions in healthcare systems*. Routledge.

Brown, H. S., & Vergragt, P. J. (2008). Bounded socio-technical experiments as agents of systemic change: The case of a zero-energy residential building. *Technological Forecasting & Social Change*, *75*(1), 107–130.

Bygherreforeningen (2021). Coronaens påvirkning af byggeprocessen [The impact of the corona virus on the construction process]. In Realdania (Ed.), *Refleksioner fra en pandemi. En essaysamling om bymiljøer, bygninger og livskvalitet i lyset af COVID-19* [Reflections from a pandemic. A collection of essays on urban environments, buildings and quality of life in the light of COVID-19] (pp. 2–3). Realdania. file:///C:/Users/jh/Downloads/Essaysamling---Refleksioner-fra-en-pandemi-FINAL%20(1).pdf

Cardona, B. (2020). The pitfalls of personalization rhetoric in time of health crisis: COVID-19 pandemic and cracks on neoliberal ideologies. *Health Promotion International*, 26(3). 10.1093/heapro/daaa112

Cherét, H. (2020). Luftforureningens høje pris. [The High Costs of Air pollution]. *Magasinet Grøn Omstilling, Vinter*, 4–6.

Clemensen, N., Dannesboe, K. I., Winther, I. W., Jordt Jørgensen, N., & Kousholt, D. (2021). Skemaer for en nedlukket hverdag [Blueprints for locked-down living]. *Dansk Paedagogisk Tidsskrift*, *2021*(2), 9–30. https://dpt.dk/temanumre/2021-2/skemaer-for-en-nedlukket-hverdag/

Dansk Erhverv. (2022). *Danskerne forventer at genoptage udlandsrejserne i 2022* [Danes expect to go abroad again in 2022]. https://www.danskerhverv.dk/siteassets/mediafolder/dokumenter/04-politik/danskerne-forventer-at-genoptage-udlandsrejserne-i-2022.pdf

Dansk Industri. (2021). *Den nye normal: 100.000 flere arbejder hjemme. DI-Analyse* [The new normal: 100 000 more people are working from home. An analysis by Danish Industry]. file:///C:/Users/jh/Downloads/Den%20nye%20normal%20-%20100.000%20flere%20arbejder%20hjemme.pdf

D'Alisa, G., & Kallis, G. (2020). Degrowth and the state. *Ecological Economics*, *169*, 106486.10.1016/j.ecolecon.2019.106486

Dryzek, J. (1997). *Politics of the earth*. Oxford University Press.

EEA. (2021). *Denmark noise fact sheet 2021*. https://www.eea.europa.eu/themes/human/noise/noise-fact-sheets/noise-country-fact-sheets-2021/denmark

Ellerman, T., Nordstrøm, C., Brandt, J., Christensen, J., Ketzel, M., Massling, A., Bossi, R., Marie Frohn, L., Geels, C., Solvang Jensen, S., Nielsen, O.-K., Winther, M., Bech Poulsen, M., Monies, C., & Sørensen, M. B. (2022). *Luftkvalitet 2020. Status for den nationale luftkvalitetsovervågning* [Air quality 2020. Status of national air quality monitoring]. Scientific Report No. 467. Danish Centre for Environment and Energy (DCE), Aarhus University. http://dce2.au.dk/pub/SR467.pdf

Engholm, I. (2023). *Design for the new world*. The University of Chicago Press.

European Union. (2022). *NextGenerationEU – make it real*. https://europa.eu/next-generation-eu/index_en

Fernando, J. W., Burden, N., Ferguson, A., O'Brien, L. V., Judge, M., & Kashima, Y. (2014). Functions of utopia: How utopian thinking motivates societal engagement. *Personality and Social Psychology Bulletin*, *44*(5). https://rest.neptune-prod.its.unimelb.edu.au/server/api/core/bitstreams/995b6df1-9c65-5e1b-a950-46f8e78af274/content

Friluftsrådet (2023, January 10). *Viden om friluftsliv og sundhed* [What we know about outdoor life and health]. Viden om friluftsliv og folkesundhed | Friluftsrådet (friluftsraadet.dk)

Frumkin, H. (2005). *Environmental health*. Jossey-Bass.
Geels, F. W. (2004). From sectoral systems of innovations to socio-technical systems. *Research Policy*, 6-7(33), 897–920.
Geels, F. W., & Kemp, R. (2012). The multi-level perspective as a new perspective for studying socio-technical transitions. In F. W. Geels, K. Rene, G. Dudley, & G. Lyons (Eds.), *Automobility in transition. A socio-technical analysis of sustainable transport* (pp. 49–79). Routledge.
Gram-Hannsen, K. (2014). Praksisteori – for en bedre forståelse af husholdningernes energiforbrug [Practice theory: For a better understanding of household energy consumption]. In J. Holm, O. Jensen, I. Stauning, & B. Søndergaard (Eds.), *Bæredygtig omstilling i bolig og byggeri* [A sustainable transition in housing and construction]. Frydenlund Academic.
Holm, J. (2022). Mod en økologisk stat? [Towards an ecological state?]. *Samfundsøkonomen*, *2022*(2), 44–57.
Holm, J., Jensen, J. O., Stauning, I., & Søndergaard, B. (Eds.) (2014). *Bæredygtig omstilling i bolig og byggeri* [A sustainable transition in housing and construction]. Frydenlund Academic.
Holm, J. & Kaae, B. (2017). *Definitionsramme for bynær økoturisme* [A definition framework for urban ecotourism]. Roskilde University. https://forskning.ruc.dk/da/publications/definitionsramme-for-b%C3%A6redygtig-byn%C3%A6r-%C3%B8koturisme
Holm, J., & Kristensen, K.A. (2014). Utopiske Levefællesskaber. [Utoipian Living Communities]. *Psyke & Logos*, *35*, 117–139.
Holm, J., Kjaergaard, B., & Jelsoe, E. (2015). Politics of co-ordination in environmental health. *Journal of Transdisciplinary Environmental Studies*, *15*(2).
IPCC (2022). Summary for policymakers. In H. O. Pörtner, D. C. Roberts, E. S. Poloczanska, K. Mintenbeck, M. Tignor, A. Alegría, M. Craig, S. Langsdorf, S. Löschke, V. Möller, & A. Okem (Eds.), *Climate change 2022: Impacts, adaptation, and vulnerability*. Contribution of Working Group II to the Sixth Assessment Report of the Intergovernmental Panel on Climate Change. Cambridge University Press. https://www.ipcc.ch/report/ar6/wg2/downloads/report/IPCC_AR6_WGII_SummaryForPolicymakers.pdf
Jacobsen, J.B. (2021). *Corona har skubbet til hvor meget magt vi tillader statenat have. [Corona have pushedthe limits for how much state intervention we may allow]. Information February12th*.
Jasanoff, S., & Kim, S.-H. (2009). Containing the atom: Sociotechnical imaginaries and nuclear power in the United States and South Korea. *Minerva*, *47*, 119–146
Jänicke, M. (1990). *State failure. The impotence of politics in industrial society*. Pennsylvania State University Press.
Jensen, S. S., Winther, M., Løfstrøm, P., & Frohn, L. M. (2019). *Kortlægning af luftforurening fra krydstogtskibe* [A survey of air pollution from cruise ships]. Scientific Report No. 316. Danish Centre for Environment and Energy (DCE), Aarhus University. http://dce2.au.dk/pub/SR316.pdf
Jessop, B. (1990). *State theory – Putting capitalist states in their place*. Polity Press
Jessop, B. (2008). *State power*. Polity Press.
Jessop, B. (2012). Economic and ecological crises: Green new deals and no-growth economies. *Development*, *55*(1), 17–24.

Jones, K., Patel, N., Levy, M., Storeygard, A., Balk, D., Gittleman, J. L., & Daszak, P. (2008). Global trends in emerging infectious diseases. *Nature*, *451*, 990–993. 10.1038/nature06536

Keesing, F., & Ostfeld, R. (2021). Impacts of biodiversity and biodiversity loss on zoonotic diseases. *Proceedings of the National Academy of Sciences*, *118*(17). 10.1073/pnas.2023540118

Kemp, R., & Rotmans, J. (2001). *The management of the co-evolution of technical, environmental and social systems*. International Conference towards Environmental Innovation Systems, Garmisch-Partenkirchen, September 2001.

Kemp, R., Schot, J., & Hoogma, R. (1998). Regime shifts to sustainability through processes of niche formation: The approach of strategic niche management. *Technology Analysis and Strategic Management*, *10*(2), 175–198.

Kemp, R., Loorbach, D., & Rotmans, J. (2007). Transition management as a model for managing processes of co-evolution towards sustainable development. *International Journal of Sustainable Development & World Ecology*, *14*, 78–91.

Koch, M. (2020). The state in the transformation to a sustainable postgrowth economy. *Environmental Politics*, *29*(1), 115–133. 10.1080/09644016.2019.1684738

Köhler, J., Geels, F. W., Kern, F., Markard, J., Onsongo, E., Wieczorek, A., Alkemade, F., Avelino, F., Bergek, A., Boons, F., Fünfschilling, L., Hess, D., Holtz, G., Hyysalo, S., Jenkins, K., Kivimaa, P., Martiskainen, M., McMeekin, A., Mühlemeier, M. S., ...Wells, P. (2019). An agenda for sustainability transitions research: State of the art and future directions. *Environmental Innovation and Societal Transitions*, *31*, 1–32. 10.1016/j.eist.2019.01.004

Latour, B. (2020, 24 April) *What protective measures can you think of so we don't go back to the pre-crisis production model?* Festival of Hope 2020, 24 April, Versopolis. https://www.versopolis.com/festival-of-hope/festival-of-hope/846/what-protective-measures-can-you-think-of-so-we-don-t-go-back-to-the-pre-crisis-production-model

Latour, B., & Schultz, N. (2022). *Notat om den nye økologiske klasse* [A note on the new ecological class]. Hans Reitzel.

Lawler, O. K., Allan, H. L., Baxter, P. W. J., Castagnino R., Tor, M. C., Dann, L. E., Hungerford J., Karmacharya, D., Lloyd, T. J., López-Jara M. J., Massie, G. N., Novera, J., Rogers, A. M., & Kark, S. (2021). The COVID-19 pandemic is intricately linked to biodiversity loss and ecosystem health. *Lancet Planet Health*. *5*(11), e840–e850.

Martell, L. (2018). Utopianism and social change: Materialism, conflict and pluralism. *Capital & Class*, 42(3), 435–452.

Meadows, D. H., Meadows, D. L., Randers, J. & Behrens, W. W. III (1972). *Limits to Growth. A REPORT FOR THE CLUB OF ROME'S PROJECT ON THE PREDICAMENT OF MANKIND*. New York: Universe Books. http://www.donellameadows.org/wp-content/userfiles/Limits-to-Growth-digital-scan-version.pdf

Mossin, N., Hinsby, P., Chevalier, T. B., Jensen, J. Z., og Vasconcelos, T. D. C. (2022). Pandemiens arkitektur [The Architecture of the pandemic]. Kunstakademiet og Realdania. file:///C:/Users/jh/Downloads/Eksempelsamling_final%20(2).pdf

Naturstyrelsen. (2020). *Vi bruger naturen mere under Corona-krisen* [We make more use of nature during the COVID-19 crisis]. https://naturstyrelsen.dk/nyheder/2020/maj/vi-bruger-naturen-mere-under-coronakrisen/

Naturstyrelsen. (2022). https://via.ritzau.dk/pressemeddelelse/naturen-er-stadig-populaer-efter-genabning?publisherId=12230032&releaseId=13645625

Nielsen, O. A., & Christiansen, H. (2021). Sådan har Corona forskudt vores transportadfærd [This is how COVID-19 has changed our transport behaviour]. In Realdania (Ed.), *Refleksioner fra en pandemi. En essaysamling om bymiljøer, bygninger og livskvalitet i lyset af COVID*-19 [Reflections from a pandemic. A collection of essays on urban environments, buildings and quality of life in the light of COVID-19] (pp. 102–114). Realdania. https://realdania.dk/publikationer/faglige-publikationer/refleksioner-fra-en-pandemi

Nygaard, B. (2014). *Håb*. Aarhus Universitet.

O'Neill, D. (2015). The proximity of nations to a socially sustainable steady-state economy. *Journal of Cleaner Production*, *108*, 1213–1231. 10.1016/j.jclepro.2015.07.116

Oomen, J., Hoffmann, K., & Hajer, M. (2022). Techniques of futuring: On how imagined futures become socially performative. *European Journal of Social Theory*, *25*(2), 252–270.

Pedersen, J. (1991). *Miljøpolitik og samfundsøkologi* [Environmental policies and social ecology]. COS Research Report No. 2. Copenhagen Business School.

Pedersen, O.K. (2020). *Vistår i politikkens øjeblik. Det er nu, vi kan forme fremtiden. [We are in the momentum of politics. It´s now wemay shape the future]*. Information May 4th.

Petersen, M. B., & Roepstorff, A. (2020, November 26). *Danskernes adfærd og holdninger til corona-epidemien.* [The Danes' behaviour and attitudes to the COVID-19 epidemic]. https://hope-project.dk/#/reports/danskernes_adfaerd_og_holdninger/versions/26-11-2020

Pichler, M., Schaffartzik, A., Haberl, H., & Görg, C. (2017). Drivers of society-nature relations in the Anthropocene and their implications for sustainability transformations. *Current Opinion in Environmental Sustainability*, *26*, 32–36. 10.1016/j.cosust.2017.01.017

Rosa, H. (2020). *Symposium – Social world and pandemic*. https://blogbvps.files.wordpress.com/2020/05/hartmut-rosa.pdf

Schultz, N., Henriksen, F. M., Blok, A., & Jacobsen, S. G. (2020). *Hvordan kan sundhedskrisen styrke den grønne omstilling?* [How can the health crisis strengthen the green transition?] Climate and Transition Council. https://www.klimaogomstillingsraadetdk/wp-content/uploads/2020/11/Corona-og-omstlling_KOR-affilieret-notat_november2020.pdf

Steffen, W., Richardson, K., Rockström, J., Cornell, S. E., Fetzer, I., Bennett, E. M., Biggs, R., Carpenter, S. R., de Vries, W., de Wit, C. A., Folke, C., Gerten, D., Heinke, J., Mace, G. M., Persson, L. M., Ramanathan, V.,Reyers, B., & Sörlin, S. (2015). Planetary boundaries: Guiding human development on a changing planet. *Science*, *347*(6223), 1259855. 10.1126/science.1259855

Toft, M., & Nielsen, A.B. (2023 forthcoming). *A Green Restart or Black to Normal? How the COVID-19 pandemic opens up a window of opportunity for the climate change policy agenda in Denmark*. Copenhagen.

UN. (2015). Transforming our world: The 2030 Agenda for Sustainable Development. Resolution adopted by the General Assembly on 25 September 2015. United Nations A/RES/70/1. [Online] Available from [Accessed 2 February 2023] http://www.un.org/ga/search/view_doc.asp?symbol=A/RES/70/1&Lang=E

UNDP. (2020). *The next frontier – Human development and the Anthropocene.* Human Development Report 2020.
Van den Broucke, S. (2020). Why health promotion matters to the COVID-19 pandemic, and vice versa. *Health Promotion International 35*(2), 181–189.
Voß, J.-P., & Kemp, R. (2006). Sustainability and reflexive governance. In J.-P. Voß, D. Bauknecht, & R. Kemp (Eds.), *Reflexive governance for sustainable development* (pp. 3–28). Edward Elgar.
WHO (2016). Shanghai Declaration on promoting health in the 2030 Agenda for Sustainable Development. 9th Global Conference on Health Pormotion, Shanghai, 21–24 November 2016. https://www.who.int/publications/i/item/WHO-NMH-PND-17.5
Willig, R., & Blok, A. (2020). *Den bæredygtige stat [The Sustainable State].* Hans Reitzelsforlag.
Wright, E. O. (2010). *Envisioning Real Utopias.* London: Verso, 2010

Part 4

Development of knowledge

Scientific changes in epidemiology and microbiology and lasting effects

12 Framing the roots of critical COVID-19 public health concepts

Intersecting history and epidemiology

Maarten van Wijhe, Søren Poder, Andreas Thomas Eilersen, and Lone Simonsen

We dedicate this chapter to our dear friend and colleague Adjunct Associate Professor Robert J Taylor who passed away recently. He made excellent contributions to the writing and content of this chapter.

We also would like to thank Mathias Mølbak Ingholt for his valuable comments and discussions during the writing of this chapter.

Introduction

Human history is marked by recurring mortality crises in the form of epidemics and pandemics. These painful lessons from the past have left a legacy in our modern public health systems. The coronavirus (COVID-19) pandemic is the latest in a long line of pandemics that have plagued societies for centuries, and our past experiences are evident in our current strategies to mitigate the impact of COVID-19: quarantine and isolation, a strong focus on hygiene, and vaccinations. Each of these pillars of pandemic response is rooted in our collective experience with infectious threats over the centuries.

In this chapter, we review the origins of three crucial COVID-19 mitigation strategies, quarantine and isolation, hygiene: and vaccination, and review their historical importance in past pandemics. Our prior experience with each of these mitigation strategies helped to shift our understanding of the management of infectious diseases in public health crises, and often represented major turning points in medical and societal development. The role of quarantine and isolation is exemplified by the plague, while cholera is known for its effect on the acceleration of the hygiene movement, and finally, vaccines can be traced back to humanity's battle against smallpox. The historical framework in conjunction with insights from modern epidemiology provides fundamental insight to reflect on the COVID-19 pandemic and how it might affect our view on these issues when, inevitably, the next pandemic, 'Disease X', emerges. We primarily use Denmark as a recurring example throughout the chapter, and in the last part, we reflect on how history shaped our

DOI: 10.4324/9781003441915-16

response to COVID-19, what we did differently, and how we might use the experience generated in modern times to prepare for the next major 'Disease X' pandemic.

Quarantines and the plague

Shunning and isolation of infected people by physical expulsion from the community dates back to antiquity, but large-scale enforcement of such measures began in earnest with the second plague pandemic, a series of bubonic plague epidemics that ran rampant through Europe from 1347 to 1723 (Snowden, 2020). Known as the Black Death, bubonic plague is an ancient disease (>6000 years old) caused by the bacterium *Yersinia pestis* (Demeure et al., 2019). Transmitted by fleas that infest rodents, especially rats, the plague probably spread along the Silk Road from the Steppes of Central Asia, via Crimea, to the Westernmost parts of Europe, the Middle East, and North Africa (Green, 2020). The most serious bubonic plague epidemic in Western history began in Messina in the Kingdom of Sicily in October 1347, from which it quickly spread to port cities such as Genoa, Barcelona, Milan, and Marseilles. Drifting along with the maritime bulk trade in grain and wool, the plague passed from one port city to the next, reaching Scandinavia and Britain in 1350. By the time the first wave ended around 1353, an astonishing 30–60% of the total European population had died of the disease (Cohn, 2017; Pradel et al., 2014). In the following centuries years, many local outbreaks of plague occurred.

Quarantines begin

The practice of imposing a period of mandatory quarantine dates back to 1377 when authorities of the Croatian city-state of Dubrovnik, located on the Adriatic coast, ordered ships arriving from plague-infected ports in the East Mediterranean to remain anchored for 40 days before landing. In practice, the period of quarantine was spent in temporary shacks erected on the outlying islands (Blažina & Blažina, 2015). However, permanent quarantine facilities originated in Venice, Italy, only two decades later. These came to lay the foundation for the European tradition of dealing with diseases such as bubonic plague.

The Venetian authorities erected two formidable quarantine facilities outside Venice on outlying islands in the lagoon: Lazzaretto Vecchio (the old hospital) and Lazzaretto Nuovo (the new hospital) were built in 1403 and 1468. Here, ships arriving from the eastern Mediterranean were required to stop. Vessels from suspect cities were carefully inspected by the legal authorities, scrubbed, and then fumigated. The crew was taken ashore under armed guard and isolated. The penalty for trying to avoid or escape quarantine was death.

Salvation in God's word

The word 'quarantine' is derived from the Italian word *quaranta*, meaning forty. In the 14th century, the choice of 40 days was not backed by any empirical evidence but strictly justified by the biblical conceptions of purification and redemption. In the Old Testament, the number 40 appears frequently in relation to God's punishment of man for his sins. The Flood lasted 40 days (Genesis 6:9–9:17), and God punished the Israelites with 40 years of wandering in the desert until the entire generation that had doubted his existence was dead (Numbers 14:34). The choice of 40 days is thus a matter of spiritual discourse: if diseases were God's punishment of men for their sins, salvation could also to be found in God's word.

In the following centuries, variations of the Venetian containment strategy became standard for combatting the plague and later cholera. For instance, European port cities such as Marseilles, Amsterdam, Rotterdam, and Copenhagen all adopted similar measures centred on a lazaretto that was either temporary or permanent, depending on the form of government and commercial interests (Baldwin, 2005; Oldstone, 2020).

In practice, most lazarettos were just temporary wooden buildings erected during times of crisis, to be either demolished or put to alternative use, often growing into institutions that dealt with broader health and social issues in the city when the epidemic threat had passed (Crawshaw, 2016; Snowden, 2020). Others were military fortifications in continuous use until the late 19th century (Crawshaw, 2016). An example of such a fortification is the fortress-like 'Il Lazzaretto', known as the Mole Vanvitelliana, which was built between 1733 and 1743 on an artificially created island in the harbour of Ancona, Italy, to protect the residents of Ancona from the plague.

Cordons sanitaires

For obvious reasons, maritime quarantine does not prevent diseases from walking through the city gates. Hence, rulers on the European mainland would in the following centuries invest considerable resources in land-based quarantine systems to block epidemics, the so-called 'cordons sanitaires' (Baldwin, 2005; Salas-Vives & Pujadas-Mora, 2018).

Like lazarettos, cordons sanitaires were meant to restrict movement of people into or out of a community, region or country. In practice, a cordon sanitaire could be a fence or wall possibly patrolled by armed troops to prevent inhabitants within the borders of the cordon from escaping, thus leaving them to battle the affliction alone. Or in the opposite case, it would prevent people from an area suspected of infection from entering a region and subsequently starting an epidemic. For example, when cholera was approaching Moscow in 1831, the Medical Council of the Ministry of the Interior in St. Petersburg was quick to place three lines of soldiers around the city and burn all but one bridge leading into the city. People who were captured trying to enter the city without permission were court-martialled and sentenced to death. Such draconian punishments were, however, exceptional and in this case partly determined by the visit of the Czar Nicholas I (1817–1855) to Moscow (Baldwin, 2005; McGrew, 1965).

Like their maritime equivalents, cordons sanitaires could be either temporary measures to combat the threat of an epidemic, or permanent and very visible militarised institutions around cities, regions or even countries (Rothenberg, 1973). Land- and maritime-based quarantines were, however, often unsuccessful in preventing a disease from entering a region in the long run. For example, the last outbreak of plague in Denmark began in the winter of 1710–1711. The autocratic monarchy had imposed a strict military blockade around the market town of Helsingør in an attempt to keep the disease away from the capital Copenhagen, 40 km to the south. However, despite quarantine measures, which interestingly excluded merchants with a travel permit, plague-infected individuals still managed to travel from Helsingør to Copenhagen, where a plague epidemic broke out in June 1711 (Frandsen, 2010). By the time the epidemic had waned, an estimated 22 000 of Copenhagen's 60 000 inhabitants had succumbed to the disease (Frandsen, 2010). If the purpose of the cordon had been to prevent the plague from spreading outside Helsingør, it failed miserably. However, it may have been successful in terms of delaying the arrival of the disease in Copenhagen.

The end of the plague

By the end of the 17th century, the plague era in Western Europe had almost come to an end. The last recorded outbreak of plague in Western Europe was in Marseilles in 1720. The blame for bringing the plague to Marseilles has been placed on the merchant vessel 'Grand Saint Antoine', which arrived in Marseilles bearing a cargo of luxurious fabrics from Smyrna and Tripoli, where plague was known to be present at the time (Devaux, 2013). When the vessel dropped anchor at the Lazaret de Saint-Martin d'Arenc outside Marseilles, eight sailors and the ship's doctor had already died at sea. The remaining crew and the vessel's cargo were according to the procedures instantly put under strict quarantine. Pressed by local merchants, however, the medical authorities agreed to release the cargo and the crew after only a shortened quarantine, and the epidemic promptly took hold. The outbreak claimed the lives of 60 000 of Marseille's 100 000 inhabitants and an additional 50 000 lives after it spread beyond the city.

It is difficult to know how effective quarantines and cordons sanitaires were in preventing or delaying the plague in spreading across Europe. What is certain is that these interventions were often subject to political, economic, and personal incentives, and therefore often imperfectly and inconsistently applied, thus diminishing their effectiveness. Economic incentives for local governments and citizens alike, as well as the substantial effort and funds required to maintain the draconian measures needed, diminished the desire to impose strict quarantine. Moreover, neither lazarettos nor cordons were non-negotiable barriers. Instead, they were imperfect measures, based in social institutions that relied on often-faulty human risk assessment. Enforcement was also bedevilled by ethnic and religious discrimination that singled out individuals or groups for strict enforcement while allowing others to travel freely (Baldwin, 2005). The impact of these interventions is difficult to assess historically, and while strict quarantine measures may have kept a disease out of a region for a time (possibly for many years, as we will see in the next section on cholera), they were often untenable and probably only delayed the disease's inevitable spread. Quarantines were mostly abandoned in Denmark as a public health measure after the first wave of cholera swept over the country in 1853; however, this was not because of their epidemiological impact, but primarily for economic reasons (Knudsen, 1988; Lützen, 2013).

Cholera and the era of hygiene as a control measure

The last quarantines enforced in Denmark before COVID-19 were in the 19th century, when cholera entered the European scene. The first cholera outbreaks in Europe were in 1831, but Denmark was spared until 1853, when a single epidemic occurred, killing 3% of the population of Copenhagen (Phelps et al., 2018). By then, cities in Germany, Sweden, and England had already suffered repeated cholera outbreaks since 1831, and the absence of cholera in Denmark before 1853 is somewhat peculiar, given the strong connections through shipping and trade. One possible factor that delayed the arrival of cholera in Denmark may have been the ship quarantine that was still imposed. The fear-induced vigilance for the disease in the medical community may also have played a role. In 1850, the young doctor Peter Panum was sent to deal with a local cholera epidemic in Bandholm, a small port in Southern Denmark. He did so successfully by improving hygiene and isolating victims, although his report and his then unconventional strategies were largely dismissed by the medical establishment (Panum, 1850). The shipping quarantine, however, was very unpopular because it interfered with trade and it was therefore abolished in 1852. The fact that a severe cholera epidemic occurred within one year of abandoning the ship quarantine certainly suggests that it may have been successful in holding the disease at bay for many years.

Whatever the reason, cholera epidemics devastated Copenhagen and other Danish towns in the autumn of 1853 (Phelps et al., 2018). Adults were particularly hard hit; in Copenhagen about one in six older people died of cholera. An outbreak usually began when an ill traveller arrived from another cholera-affected area, typically by ship (Holst, 1859; Panum, 1850). Patients were often tended to by locals who would fall ill after a few days and bring the disease to their household, thus starting an outbreak. A similar epidemic pattern was observed in towns and cities, regardless of water source (piped water, rivers, or local pumps). This suggested that cholera was not only water-borne, but also spread from person to person through contact with, e.g., contaminated waste and clothing (Phelps, 2018). Thus ship quarantines, isolation, and improved hygiene measures were likely to have been effective by limiting the risk of arrival of infected travellers and by preventing further spread through contaminated surfaces, goods, and drinking water.

Cholera as an urban crisis

Cholera came to highlight the social costs of 19th-century urbanisation and industrialisation, which transformed centuries-old socioeconomic institutions and became a defining crisis of modern European societies (Friedrichs, 1995; De Vries, 2013). The industrial revolution was a far-reaching transformation of society in Western European and North America; it started in England in the mid-18th century and lasted until the early 20th century. This was a time of innovation, progress, and rapid growth of towns and cities. However, it was also often accompanied by increased poverty in the working class (Hamlin et al., 1998). A 12-hour workday in dark and unventilated factories was normal for adults as well as children; in the 19th century, child labour was common and crucial for the early industrial economies (Humphries, 2010). The need for workforces resulted in increasing urbanisation, rapidly growing towns, and increasing population densities.

During this time, production became considerably more effective and transportation times were greatly reduced, improving the interconnectivity of countries and cities, and erasing previous barriers to international trade (Andersen et al., 2005; Hohenberg & Lees, 1995). For instance, the Suez Canal opened in 1859, reducing travel time from England to India from months to just nine weeks. However, high-density living, poor hygiene, and lack of proper nutrition, combined with rapid population movement, created the ideal setting for infectious diseases to spread. For example, the construction of a network of railways meant that people could travel over long distances well within the short incubation period of cholera: a person could board a train in perfect health and a day later arrive with full-blown infectious cholera in another city or country (Azman et al., 2013). Thus, urbanisation and increased connectivity gave rise to societies that were highly susceptible to diseases such as cholera.

The rise of sanitation

Ship quarantines were never reintroduced in Denmark. This may have been due to the dramatically changed beliefs about cholera infectivity. In 1831, cholera was understood to be a contagious disease that could be controlled by isolation and quarantine, while the dominant point of view around 1853 was that cholera was transmitted by 'miasma' emanating from swamps and sewers (Sommer, 1854). In this perspective, isolation and quarantine made less sense because the disease was caused by miasmas that were already present, lurking in the filth of the local environment. But perspectives were changing. The miasma theory receded later in the century when the microbiology era yielded clear evidence of an infectious disease paradigm, when Robert Koch and colleagues demonstrated that the disease was caused by *Vibrio cholerae*, a gram-negative bacteria that spreads via the oral-faecal route.

The deadly cholera epidemics of the 19th century and the changing paradigm made doctors increasingly aware of the importance of living conditions and population health measures such as waste management, hygiene, and clean drinking water. Rapid urbanisation required action to improve city planning and infrastructure. In Denmark, cholera accelerated this movement, spearheaded by key physicians who went into politics to improve the health of the population. The late 19th century saw a dramatic decline in infectious disease mortality, with an especially steep reduction in paediatric deaths (Løkke, 1998). Improved chances of surviving early childhood, especially in urban environments, led to dramatic increases in life expectancy at birth, which increased in Denmark from around 40 years in 1850 to 50 years by 1900 and 60 years by 1925. The exact reasons for the decline in mortality and the contribution of improvements in hygiene are still subject to debate.

In Denmark and other European countries, this modern paradigm and the resulting focus on epidemic prevention also led to the introduction and extension of legislation on epidemics that gave governments extensive powers in the case of an epidemic or pandemic crisis. In Denmark, these laws built upon a previous law from 1782, which was aimed solely at rural areas, and included mandates such as preventing large gatherings, restrictions on rituals during burials, and quarantines. It was extended and amended several times (in 1831, 1888, 1893, and 1915), often extending the powers of the authorities in epidemic situations. The final amendment came after more than a century, when it was reviewed in 2020 due to the COVID-19 pandemic.

Smallpox and the beginning of vaccination programmes

Smallpox is an infectious disease caused by the variola virus. There are two main variants of this virus, *Variola major* and *Variola minor*, of which *V. major* causes the more severe illness (Dumbell et al., 1961; van Campenhout, 1935). The virus is an exclusively human pathogen which has afflicted humankind for thousands of years. Although its origins are disputed, evidence points to a zoonotic origin, possibly coming from an African rodent virus during the Paleolithic era (Li et al., 2007). Smallpox was endemic to most of the world for many centuries and caused up to one-eighth of all mortality in Europe in the mid-18th century (Baxby, 1999), with an observed case fatality rate of 17% in one early 20th-century outbreak (Albert et al., 2001).

Because smallpox was such a deadly disease, there was considerable interest in any means to treat it or mitigate its spread. In the 18th century, variolation was one such preventative measure. However, this method was quite dangerous and entailed deliberate infection with a small dose of infectious material from a person with smallpox, usually from a scab, by inhaling a powdered form or by insertion under the skin. By the end of the 18th century, it was noted that milkmaids who had previously been infected with cowpox rarely seemed to contract smallpox, indicating that zoonotic infection with cowpox, a smallpox-like disease of cattle, provided protection (Barquet & Domingo, 1997). Some people, such as Peter Plett, had already around 1790 recognised the potential of the typically mild cowpox infection to protect against smallpox, but their discoveries were largely ignored (Plett, 2006).

Jenner, an English doctor, was the first to systematically test the prophylactic effect of cowpox inoculation against smallpox. He inoculated people who had previously had cowpox with live smallpox material. The test subjects displayed few to no symptoms. He proceeded to inoculate several local children with cowpox, and after their recovery exposed some of them to smallpox. None of the children developed any significant symptoms. These findings were published in his 1798 book, *Inquiry into the Causes and Effects of the Variolae Vaccinae* (Jenner, 1798). Cowpox inoculation thus became the world's first vaccine.

Vaccination programmes

The new vaccine immediately caused ripples throughout the world. Where variolation had been risky, the cowpox-based vaccine promised to have fewer problems. Initially, however, the vaccine did not quite live up to this promise. Rare side effects included an uncontrolled generalised infection and encephalitis, both of which could be fatal (Belongia & Naleway, 2003). Before the formulation of the germ theory of disease, propagation of the vaccine from arm to arm with non-sterile equipment was common, resulting in transmission of syphilis and other blood-borne diseases.

Regardless of these issues, vaccination was safer than variolation and Jenner's vaccine was very soon generally adopted in Europe. For example, as early as in 1801 more than 100 000 children had been vaccinated in England, and by 1810, 70% of Danish children had received the vaccination. With such a sudden introduction of a new medical practice to the general population, it was hardly surprising that resistance arose, and an incipient anti-vaccine movement formed (Bonderup, 2001). This was driven in part by a general public scepticism of the growing power of doctors in 19th-century society. Scepticism intensified greatly as vaccine mandates were put into place, such as the English 1853 requirement for all parents to have their children vaccinated or face fines (Brunton, 2008). Many cast doubt on the efficacy and safety of the vaccine, and often philosophical beliefs about health and healing played a role in resistance to vaccination (Wolfe & Sharp, 2002). One important legacy of vaccine resistance has been the introduction of 'conscientious objector' clauses in vaccine mandates and similar laws in many countries (Wolfe & Sharp, 2002). In Denmark, it has been argued that the mandatory smallpox vaccination that began in 1810 represented the beginnings of the country's tradition of (semi-)voluntary participation in public health programmes (Bonderup, 2001). Scientifically, the success of the smallpox vaccine paved the way for the emergence of a new medical field.

Breakthroughs in microbiology in the late 19th century led to a burst of new discoveries on vaccines. In 1879, Louis Pasteur by chance observed that laboratory cultivation could attenuate formerly virulent bacterial cultures, a discovery he then used to create a vaccine against chicken cholera, an economically devastating disease. This vaccine was the first ever to be developed in a laboratory (Plotkin, 1996). The new method eventually led to the development of vaccines against tuberculosis (BCG), measles, and other diseases. Emil von Behring developed the first toxoid-based vaccines, which provided immunity to a bacterial toxin instead of the bacterium itself. These included his vaccine against diphtheria in 1913, a major cause of mortality in children at the time (Burkovski, 2014). The modern development of live-attenuated vaccines against paediatric diseases such as measles, mumps, and rubella in the 1960s was enabled by cell culture methods developed in the early 20th century. Subunit vaccines and new methods of synthesis came in the late 20th century, but few major breakthroughs resulted (Hilleman, 2000). Finally, in the early 1990s, the first steps were taken towards the mRNA vaccine technology[1] that came to prominence during the COVID-19 pandemic (Verbeke et al., 2019). Although a great deal has changed in the past 200 years of vaccine history, we owe today's record-breaking pace of vaccine development during COVID-19 to a series of scientific advances which can be traced back to the first observations of cowpox-induced immunity against smallpox.

COVID-19 perspectives

When the first wave of the COVID-19 pandemic spread around the world in 2020, we employed age-old strategies like quarantine, isolation, and hygiene measures to slow down its initial spread while the world waited for vaccines to be developed and distributed. These strategies have a long history, stemming from our collective experience from previous epidemics and pandemics. In this section, we use this historical perspective to reflect on the COVID-19 pandemic, with particular attention to the Danish experience.

'Lockdowns' (a more modern word for extensive quarantine measures) were quickly mandated in the first months of the COVID-19 pandemic when it became clear that hospitals would not be able to cope with the numbers of severely ill patients if COVID-19 was to propagate freely. In Denmark, mitigation strategies, including the stringency of lockdowns, were continuously revised based on mathematical model-based estimates of hospital admissions. The main objective was to control the disease enough to keep the number of patients admitted to hospitals within the capacity of the health system. The notion of slowing down rather than stopping or preventing the outbreak stands in contrast to the overall historical use of quarantine and isolation, which aimed, but often failed, to keep an infectious disease out of a healthy population.

Like many countries in Europe, Denmark went into lockdown in mid-March 2020. It was the first time since the 1892 cholera outbreak in Hamburg that borders were (partially) closed due to a disease outbreak. Physical distancing became the norm, public employees were advised or ordered to work remotely, and educational institutions were required to conduct remote teaching. Non-essential stores, bars, restaurants, concerts, and amusement parks were ordered to close, and nursing homes were closed to visitors to prevent the introduction of infection into the older population (SKR Nr 9161, 2020). Despite the historical evidence of the unsustainability of strict quarantines, some governments, as in China and Australia, embarked on a 'zero-COVID' strategy, instituting long-term strict lockdowns and border closures that aimed to keep society completely COVID-free. In the short term, they were successful, and indeed Australia managed to exit its zero-COVID era with a highly vaccinated population in autumn 2021. Meanwhile, China's 'zero-COVID' strategy started to fail in April 2022 despite strict quarantines and in December 2022, China officially ended its lockdown measures after continued public protests. The country was immediately subject to an unmitigated epidemic wave (Dyer, 2022; Ioannidis et al., 2023). Whether this zero-COVID strategy of strict quarantines paid off in terms of reduced mortality or economic consequences remains to be evaluated.

Governments were also quick to enforce personal hygiene guidelines such as frequent disinfection of hands and surfaces, the use of facemasks, and improved ventilation. The hygiene movement of the 19th century took place against the backdrop of the miasma paradigm and focused mainly on structural and sanitation changes in cities spurred on by the cholera outbreaks of the time. While the reasoning behind these measures changed with the shift in the second half of the 19th century from a miasma way of thinking to a contagion perspective, the idea of enforcing hygiene measures and improving sanitation infrastructure has remained a key tool to control infectious diseases. The personal hygiene measures strongly emphasised during COVID-19 stem from the same paradigm shift and focus on minimising person-to-person spread. While some agents, such as influenza virus and pathogens transmitted through the oral-faecal route, can effectively be controlled by washing hands and disinfection of surfaces, airborne agents are more effectively mitigated by ventilation and face masks (Wang et al., 2022). The role of personal hygiene measures during the COVID-19 pandemic was heavily discussed. Initially, SARS-CoV-2 was thought to spread through contaminated surfaces, and despite early evidence of airborne spread, this notion held for nearly two years (Wang et al., 2022). However, although some of the hygiene measures employed may not have been the most effective against SARS-CoV-2, they are generally advisable and may also have contributed to the disappearance of influenza during the pandemic (Huang et al., 2021).

The COVID-19 pandemic was the first in history where in many countries quarantine and isolation were consciously used to slow disease spread; it was also the first pandemic to be controlled by vaccination. Since smallpox, vaccination has been a cornerstone in our fight against many childhood infectious diseases. When COVID-19 emerged, it placed new requirements on vaccine development. If the vaccine were to be of any use during the pandemic, it had to be developed within a short space of time. The previous record for vaccine development time was four years for the mumps vaccine (Buynak & Hilleman, 1966). The extremely expedited development of COVID-19 vaccines was achieved by running phase II and III clinical trials concurrently, and enrolling unprecedented numbers of volunteers in the trials (Falsey et al., 2021; Oliver et al., 2020). Furthermore, the first approved vaccines (Pfizer/BioNTech, Moderna, AstraZeneca, and Johnson & Johnson) were all based on novel technologies that had already shown promising safety data in previous research (Verbeke et al., 2019). Specifically, mRNA and viral vector vaccines had the additional advantage that they could relatively easily be modified to fit a new pathogen (Custers et al., 2021) See endnoteq. Another change to expedite vaccine development was parallel production. Likely vaccine candidates were already on the production line with strong governmental support before the outcome of phase three clinical trials and approval were finalised (Kuter et al., 2021). This meant that millions of doses were ready for distribution within a short time after approval. The timely implementation of vaccination strategies changed perspectives on COVID-19 and the aim of other control strategies; vaccination became 'the way out of the pandemic'.

The COVID-19 pandemic not only offered a challenge for vaccine development, but also for public acceptance of vaccination. The rapid development of several different vaccines, their initial scarcity and uncertain effectiveness and risk profiles, together with the continually changing guidelines necessitated by the evolving virus, made it difficult to provide clear communication about vaccinations to the public. Denmark, like other countries, faced vocal groups opposing vaccination and other mitigation strategies. In some settings, vaccine hesitation led to unfortunate outcomes. One example is Bulgaria, where despite access to vaccines only about 30% of the population was vaccinated at the start of 2022. This, combined with poor epidemic control, led to the deaths from COVID-19 of an estimated 1% of the population (Mathieu et al., 2023). The phenomenon of vaccine hesitation is not new, but goes back to the introduction of smallpox vaccination and is also seen in other modern vaccination programmes. One difference between today's vaccine resistance and its historical roots is the degree of organisation and vociferousness made possible by social media and other modern communication tools (Yaqub et al., 2014). Nonetheless, support for SARS-CoV-2 mass vaccination programmes has been strong in most Western countries (Gramacho & Turgeon, 2021; Mathieu et al., 2021). The distribution of vaccinations has also been criticised for being discriminatory, with wealthy countries quickly buying up available stockpiles, leaving little for the rest of the world. In the globalised society, these examples put stress on governments that are hard-pressed to find a balance between serving the interests of their own populations and philanthropic expectations (Iserson, 2021).

Concluding remarks

With each pandemic event, we are forced to rely on what we have learned from past pandemics and build upon that knowledge. In the last century, growing medical optimism repeatedly held that infectious diseases would soon be forgotten relics of earlier times. First came the understanding that microorganisms caused disease, then came laboratory-developed vaccines, and later antibiotics. Optimism peaked with the eradication of smallpox. Unfortunately, that optimism has faded in the face of new pathogenic threats such as the HIV, H5N1 influenza, SARS, Zika, and Ebola. To this list, we can now add SARS-CoV-2, and it will not be the last to be added. In 2018, the WHO placed the so-called 'Disease X' on their list of *blueprint priority diseases*, that is, diseases which are likely to cause future public health emergencies, and which require increased vigilance. The COVID-19 pandemic revitalised the focus on pandemic preparedness and made us aware that Disease X, the new deadly global threat, remains ever on the horizon. Yet we learn lessons from every new pandemic event. Our response to COVID-19 was the culmination of our collective past pandemic experience. The major new developments, which will surely also help us to combat the next pandemic, were the central role of mathematical modelling to inform decision making and the pivotal role of vaccinations to finally control the pandemic. But old lessons die hard, and mistrust persists, both with regard to whether the hardships of mitigation were worth it, and vaccine hesitancy, which remains a major obstacle in some settings.

COVID-19 has reminded us of the importance of pandemic preparedness and the constant threat of new diseases. Our response to COVID-19 has taught us valuable lessons and led to important advances, including finding a new purpose for data-driven traditional mitigation strategies that helped to overcome the initial pandemic phase while vaccines were being developed. As we move forward and remain vigilant for Disease X, it will be important to continue building on these achievements, while heeding the lessons from our past experiences.

Note

1 The mRNA vaccine technology differs from earlier vaccine types by relying on messenger RNA. Messenger RNA is bits of genetic code from the pathogen that stimulate dendritic immune cells to presentantigens of the pathogen on their surface, thus training the immune system to recognize the pathogen. mRNA vaccines are relatively easily tailored to new pathogens by exchanging mRNA components.

References

Albert, M. R., Ostheimer, K. G., & Breman, J. G. (2001). The last smallpox epidemic in Boston and the vaccination controversy, 1901–1903. *New England Journal of Medicine*, *344*(5), 375–379. 10.1056/NEJM200102013440511

Andersen, H. T., Christensen, S. B., Dragsbo, P., Jensen, J. T., Knudsen, K., Nielsen, B., Pedersen, M. B., Pinholt, N. H., Sommer, A.-L., Thelle, M., Ladegaard, M., Tofte, U., & Thøgersen, M. (2005). *Den moderne by* [The modern city] (S. B. Christensen, Ed.). Aarhus University Press.

Azman, A. S., Rudolph, K. E., Cummings, D. A. T., & Lessler, J. (2013). The incubation period of cholera: A systematic review. *The Journal of Infection*, *66*(5), 432–438. 10.1016/j.jinf.2012.11.013

Baldwin, P. (2005). *Contagion and the state in Europe, 1830–1930*. Cambridge University Press.

Barquet, N., & Domingo, P. (1997). Smallpox: The triumph over the most terrible of the ministers of death. *Annals of Internal Medicine*, *127*(8_Part_1), 635–642. 10.7326/0003-4819-127-8_Part_1-199710150-00010

Baxby, D. (1999). Edward Jenner's inquiry: A bicentenary analysis. *Vaccine*, *17*(4), 301–307. 10.1016/S0264-410X(98)00207-2

Belongia, E. A., & Naleway, A. L. (2003). Smallpox vaccine: The good, the bad, and the ugly. *Clinical Medicine & Research*, *1*(2), 87–92. 10.3121/CMR.1.2.87

Blažina, Z. T., & Blažina, V. (2015). *Expelling the plague: The health office and implementation of quarantine in Dubrovnik, 1377–1533*. McGill-Queens University Press.

Bonderup, G. (2001). *En kovending: koppevaccinationen og dens udfordring til det danske samfund omkring 1800* [A u-turn: Smallpox vaccination and its challenge for Danish society around 1800]. Aarhus University Press.

Brunton, D. (2008). *The politics of vaccination: Practice and policy in England, Wales, Ireland, and Scotland, 1800–1874*. University of Rochester Press.

Burkovski, A. (2014). Diphtheria and its etiological agents. In A. Burkovski (Ed.), *Corynebacterium diphtheriae and related toxigenic species: Genomics, pathogenicity and applications* (pp. 1–14). Springer. 10.1007/978-94-007-7624-1_1

Buynak, E. B., & Hilleman, M. R. (1966). Live attenuated mumps virus vaccine. 1. Vaccine development. *Proceedings of the Society for Experimental Biology and Medicine*, *123*(3), 768–775. 10.3181/00379727-123-31599

Cohn, S. K. (2017). The black death: The end of a paradigm. In J. Canning, H. Lehmann, & J. M. Winter (Eds.), *Power, violence and mass death in pre-modern and modern times* (pp. 25–66). Ashgate. 10.4324/9781315246253-4

Crawshaw, J. L. S. (2016). *Plague hospitals: Public health for the city in early modern Venice*. Routledge.

Custers, J., Kim, D., Leyssen, M., Gurwith, M., Tomaka, F., Robertson, J., Heijnen, E., Condit, R., Shukarev, G., Heerwegh, D., van Heesbeen, R., Schuitemaker, H., Douoguih, M., Evans, E., Smith, E. R., & Chen, R. T. (2021). Vaccines based on replication incompetent Ad26 viral vectors: Standardized template with key considerations for a risk/benefit assessment. *Vaccine*, *39*(22), 3081–3101. 10.1016/J.VACCINE.2020.09.018

Demeure, C., Dussurget, O., Fiol, G. M., Le Guern, A. S., Savin, C., & Pizarro-Cerdá, J. (2019). Yersinia pestis and plague: An updated view on evolution, virulence determinants, immune subversion, vaccination and diagnostics. *Microbes and Infection*, *21*(5-6), 202–212. 10.1016/j.micinf.2019.06.007

Devaux, C. A. (2013). Small oversights that led to the Great Plague of Marseille (1720–1723): Lessons from the past. *Infection, Genetics and Evolution*, *14*(1), 169–185. 10.1016/j.meegid.2012.11.016

De Vries, J. (2013). *European urbanization, 1500–1800*. Routledge.

Dumbell, K. R., Bedson, H. S., & Rossier, E. (1961). The laboratory differentiation between variola major and variola minor. *Bulletin of the World Health Organization*, *25*, 73–78.

Dyer, O. (2022). Covid-19: Lockdowns spread in China as omicron tests "zero covid" strategy. *British Medical Journal*, *376*, o859. 10.1136/bmj.o859

Falsey, A. R., Sobieszczyk, M. E., Hirsch, I., Sproule, S., Robb, M. L., Corey, L., Neuzil, K. M., Hahn, W., Hunt, J., Mulligan, M. J., McEvoy, C., DeJesus, E., Hassman, M., Little, S. J., Pahud, B. A., Durbin, A., Pickrell, P., Daar, E. S., Bush, L., …Gonzalez-Lopez, A. (2021). Phase 3 safety and efficacy of AZD1222 (ChAdOx1 nCoV-19) Covid-19 vaccine. *New England Journal of Medicine*, *385*(25), 2348–2360. 10.1056/NEJMOA2105290/SUPPL_FILE/NEJMOA2105290_DATA-SHARING.PDF

Frandsen, K.-E. (2010). *Last plague in the Baltic region, 1709–1713*. Museum Tusculanum Press.

Friedrichs, C. (1995). *The early modern city, 1450–1750 (A history of urban society in Europe)*. Longman.

Gramacho, W. G., & Turgeon, M. (2021). When politics collides with public health: COVID-19 vaccine country of origin and vaccination acceptance in Brazil. *Vaccine*, *39*(19), 2608–2612. 10.1016/J.VACCINE.2021.03.080

Green, M. H. (2020). The four black deaths. *The American Historical Review*, *125*(5), 1601–1631.

Hamlin, C., Press, C. U., Jones, C., Rosenberg, C., & Jones, P. E. H. C. (1998). *Public health and social justice in the age of Chadwick: Britain, 1800–1854*. Cambridge University Press.

Hilleman, M. R. (2000). Vaccines in historic evolution and perspective: A narrative of vaccine discoveries. *Vaccine*, *18*(15), 1436–1447. 10.1016/S0264-410X(99)00434-X

Hohenberg, P. M., & Lees, L. H. (1995). *The making of urban Europe, 1000–1994*. Harvard University Press.

Holst, E. (1859). *Meddelelser om koleraepidemien i Korsör i 1857: især i hygienjnisk og statistisk henseende, samt bidrag til en medicinsk topographi af Korsör, en afhandling for doktorgraden i medicinen* [Notifications of the cholera epidemic in Korsör in 1857]. Otto Schwartz.

Huang, Q. S., Wood, T., Jelley, L., Jennings, T., Jefferies, S., Daniells, K., Nesdale, A., Dowell, T., Turner, N., Campbell-Stokes, P., Balm, M., Dobinson, H. C., Grant, C. C., James, S., Aminisani, N., Ralston, J., Gunn, W., Bocacao, J., Danielewicz, J., ... NPIsImpactOnFlu Consortium (2021). Impact of the COVID-19 nonpharmaceutical interventions on influenza and other respiratory viral infections in New Zealand. *Nature Communications*, *12*(1), 1001. 10.1038/s41467-021-21157-9

Humphries, J. (2010). *Childhood and child labour in the British industrial revolution*. Cambridge University Press. 10.1017/CBO9780511780455

Ioannidis, J. P. A., Zonta, F., & Levitt, M. (2023). Estimates of COVID-19 deaths in Mainland China after abandoning zero COVID policy. *European Journal of Clinical Investigation*, e13956. 10.1111/eci.13956

Iserson, K. (2021). SARS-CoV-2 (COVID-19) vaccine development and production: An ethical way forward. *Cambridge Quarterly of Healthcare Ethics*, *30*(1), 59–68. 10.1017/S096318012000047X

Jenner, E. (1798). *An inquiry into the causes and effects of the variolae vaccinae, a disease discovered in some of the western counties of England, particularly Gloucestershire, and known by the name of the cow pox*. Sampson Low.

Knudsen, T. (1988). *Storbyen støbes. København mellem kaos og byplan 1840–1917*. [The city is forged. Copenhagen between chaos and urban planning 1840–1917]. Akademisk Forlag.

Kuter, B. J., Offit, P. A., & Poland, G. A. (2021). The development of COVID-19 vaccines in the United States: Why and how so fast? *Vaccine*, *39*(18), 2491–2495. 10.1016/j.vaccine.2021.03.077

Li, Y., Carroll, D. S., Gardner, S. N., Walsh, M. C., Vitalis, E. A., & Damon, I. K. (2007). On the origin of smallpox: Correlating variola phylogenics with historical smallpox records. *Proceedings of the National Academy of Sciences of the United States of America*, *104*(40), 15787–15792. 10.1073/PNAS.0609268104

Løkke, A. (1998). *Døden i barndommen. Spædbørnsdødlighed og moderniseringsprocesser i Danmark 1800–1920*. [Death in childhood. Infant mortality and modernization in Denmark 1800–1920]. Gyldendal.

Lützen, K. C. (2013). *Byen Tæmmes - kernefamilie, sociale reformer og velgørenhed i 1800-tallets København* [Taming the city: The nuclear family, social reforms and charitable work in 19th century Copenhagen] (2nd ed.). Gyldendal.

Mathieu, E., Ritchie, H., Ortiz-Ospina, E., Roser, M., Hasell, J., Appel, C., Giattino, C., & Rodés-Guirao, L. (2021). A global database of COVID-19 vaccinations. *Nature Human Behaviour*, *5*(7), 947–953. 10.1038/s41562-021-01122-8

Mathieu, E., Ritchie, H., Rodés-Guirao, L., Appel, C., Giattino, C., Hasell, J., Macdonald, B., Dattani, S., Beltekian, D., Ortiz-Ospina, E., & Roser, M. (2023). *Coronavirus pandemic (COVID-19)*. Our world in data. https://ourworldindata.org/coronavirus

McGrew, R. E. (1965). *Russia and the cholera, 1823–32*. University of Wisconsin Press.

Oldstone, M. B. (2020). *Viruses, plagues, and history: Past, present, and future*. Oxford University Press.

Oliver, S. E., Gargano, J. W., Marin, M., Wallace, M., Curran, K. G., Chamberland, M., McClung, N., Campos-Outcalt, D., Morgan, R. L., Mbaeyi, S., Romero, J. R., Talbot, H. K., Lee, G. M., Bell, B. P., & Dooling, K. (2020). The Advisory

Committee on Immunization Practices' interim recommendation for use of Pfizer-BioNTech COVID-19 Vaccine – United States, December 2020. *Morbidity and Mortality Weekly Report*, *69*(50), 1922. 10.15585/MMWR.MM6950E2

Panum, P. L. (1850). *Om Cholera-Epidemien i Bandholm 1850* [About the cholera epidemic in Bandholm 1850]. Bianco Luno.

Phelps, M., Perner, M. L., Pitzer, V. E., Andreasen, V., Jensen, P. K. M., & Simonsen, L. (2018). Cholera epidemics of the past offer new insights into an old enemy. *Journal of Infectious Diseases*, *217*(4). 10.1093/infdis/jix602

Plett, P. C. (2006). Peter Plett and other discoverers of cowpox vaccination before Edward Jenner. *Sudhoffs Archiv*, *90*(2), 219–232.

Plotkin, S. A. (1996). A hundred years of vaccination: The legacy of Louis Pasteur. *The Pediatric Infectious Disease Journal*, *15*(5), 391–394.

Pradel, E., Lemaître, N., Merchez, M., Ricard, I., Reboul, A., Dewitte, A., & Sebbane, F. (2014). New insights into how Yersinia pestis adapts to its mammalian host during bubonic plague. *PLoS Pathogens*, *10*(3). 10.1371/journal.ppat.1004029

Rothenberg, G. E. (1973). The Austrian sanitary cordon and the control of the bubonic plague: 1710–1871. *Journal of the History of Medicine and Allied Sciences*, *28*(1), 15–23.

Salas-Vives, P., & Pujadas-Mora, J. M. (2018). Cordons sanitaires and the rationalisation process in Southern Europe (nineteenth-century Majorca). *Medical History*, *62*(3), 314–332. 10.1017/mdh.2018.25

Social- og Indenrigsministeriet. Orientering om forsamlingsforbud, besøgsrestriktioner og hjemgivelse af anbragte børn og unge [Orientation on assembly bans, visitor restrictions and repatriation of children and young people placed in care]. SKR Nr 9161, Pub. L. No. 225484 (2020).

Snowden, F. M. (2020). *Epidemics and society: From the black death to the present*. Yale University Press.

Sommer, A. (1854). Cholera's Udbredelsesmaade i Kongeriget Danmark (med Undtagels af Kjöbenhavn) i Aaret 1853 [The method of transmission of cholera in the Kingdom of Denmark (with the exception of Copenhagen) in the year 1853]. *Bibliotek for Læger*, *14*, 286–377.

van Campenhout, E. (1935). *The diagnosis of variola major and variola minor*. Bulletin de l'Office International d'Hygiene.

Verbeke, R., Lentacker, I., De Smedt, S. C., & Dewitte, H. (2019). Three decades of messenger RNA vaccine development. *Nano Today*, *28*, 100766. 10.1016/J.NANTOD.2019.100766

Wang, C. C., Prather, K. A., Sznitman, J., Jimenez, J. L., Lakdawala, S. S., Tufekci, Z., & Marr, L. C. (2022). Airborne transmission of respiratory viruses. *Science*, *373*(6558), eabd9149. 10.1126/science.abd9149

Wolfe, R. M., & Sharp, L. K. (2002). Anti-vaccinationists past and present. *British Medical Journal*, *325*(7361), 430–432. 10.1136/BMJ.325.7361.430

Yaqub, O., Castle-Clarke, S., Sevdalis, N., & Chataway, J. (2014). Attitudes to vaccination: A critical review. *Social Science and Medicine*, *112*, 1–11. 10.1016/j.socscimed.2014.04.018

13 The gut feeling during the COVID-19 pandemic

Hengameh Chloé Mirsepasi-Lauridsen, Camilla Adler Sørensen, Jesper Thorvald Troelsen, and Karen Angeliki Krogfelt

Introduction

Early descriptions characterised viruses as filterable agents that could pass through filters that retained bacteria. This led to the notion that viruses were smaller than bacteria, and they were often described as submicroscopic particles. Since viruses were not able to grow or reproduce outside of living cells, they were often considered to be a type of poison or toxin. In the early 20th century, it was demonstrated that viruses were composed of genetic material, either DNA or RNA, and protein. This led to the understanding that viruses were not simply toxins, but rather complex biological entities with their own unique properties. As research into viruses continued, scientists refined their understanding of these entities, recognising their ability to infect and hijack host cells to replicate and cause disease. Today, viruses are recognised as a major cause of disease in humans and other organisms and continue to be the subject of ongoing research and discovery. Viruses are the leading edge of the evolution of all living entities, as they have been for 1.5 billion years, and they must no longer be left out of the tree of life, thanks to modern technology and knowledge gained about viruses in the last century (Villarreal, 2005).

The intruders

Most well-studied human viruses are pathogenic (Villarreal, 2005). There are over 200 viral species that are known to infect humans and cause epidemics such as yellow fever in 1901 (Gardner & Ryman, 2010), the 'Spanish flu' in 1918, by the H1N1 influenza virus, the Severe Acute Respiratory Syndrome coronavirus 1 (SARS-CoV-1) in 2002, Ebola viruses in 2014 (Beaven, 2004) and SARS-CoV-2 virus in 2020 (Abdolmaleki et al., 2022; Yang et al., 2020a). Human viruses infect human cells (Villarreal, 2005), and most human viruses can also infect animals, and viruses that infect animals can jump back to humans (Ellwanger & Chies, 2021; Villarreal, 2005).

That was the case with Ebola virus and SARS, that were circulating in bats and other animals. Once a virus enters a new host cell, it must interact with

DOI: 10.4324/9781003441915-17

hundreds of proteins to complete its life cycle, while evading the new host's immune system and simultaneously induce changes in the virus genome. When a virus is spreading among animals and occasionally jumps back to humans, it is known as zoonotic spillover, which poses its own threats to public health (Ellwanger & Chies, 2021) (Figure 13.1).

Coronaviruses are named 'corona' because of their crown-like spikes on the surfaces of the virus. Coronaviruses are a family of viruses that can cause respiratory illness such as SARS and the common cold (Dimmock et al., 2016). Coronaviruses exist in, e.g., bats, cats, and camels without causing infection, but they can cause severe infection when transmitted to humans. The SARS-CoV-1 outbreak in 2002–2004 originated at a food market in China, where people were infected through contact with meat, fish and live animals such as bats (Yang et al., 2020a; Zhang et al., 2020a). SARS-CoV-1 spread to 32 different countries/regions in 2002–2003, infected 8422 people,

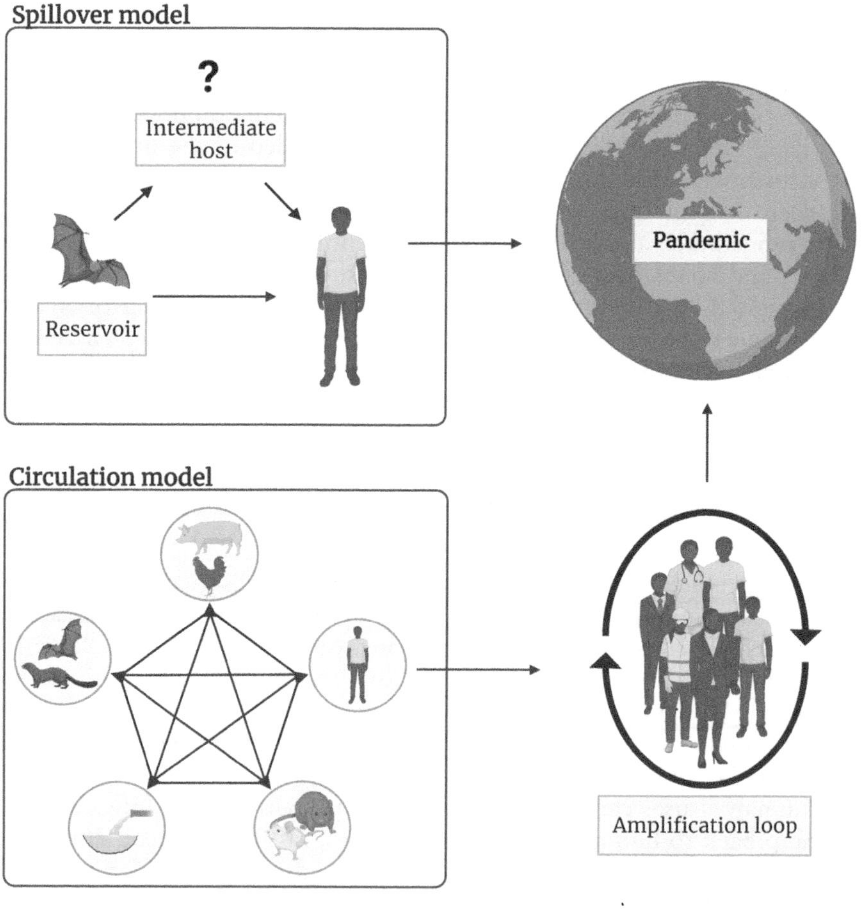

Figure 13.1 Schematic model of disease transmission in the population.

and caused 919 SARS-related deaths (Yang et al., 2020b). In late December 2019, SARS-CoV-2, a new strain of coronavirus closely related to SARS-CoV-1, was discovered in Wuhan, China. SARS-CoV-2 appeared to be milder, but with 10–20 times higher binding affinity than SARS-CoV-1, causing more efficient cell entry (Abdolmaleki et al., 2022; Yang et al. 2020b), and much faster spreading among humans. Within a short time, SARS-CoV-2 became a pandemic, not only causing severe respiratory illness, but also affecting other human organs such as the heart and gut, causing severe disease in older individuals and those with autoimmune/chronic disease (Fekadu et al., 2021).

However, not all viruses cause disease in the human body. There are millions of beneficial microorganisms, i.e., viruses/phages, bacteria, fungi, and parasites, covering our body inside and outside (Sender et al., 2016). The human ecosystem consists of 43% human cells and 57% foreign cells/microorganisms, which play an essential role for human health by degrading food to nutrients and vitamins, protecting us against infection, and by providing essential health benefits though maturation of our immune system and regulation of immune homeostasis (Sender et al., 2016).

The first and most essential colonisation process of the human body with microorganisms starts through the birth canal, where the new-born receives the mother's microbiota (Mueller et al., 2015). Thereafter, environment, diet, living conditions, and usage of antibiotics play an essential role to shape our body's microorganisms as we grow older. The composition of microorganisms is unique to each person, like a 'fingerprint' (Figure 13.2). The gastrointestinal tract is a very complex environment, where it is vital that bacteria grow and multiply in balance with the intestinal cells and the immune system (Sender et al., 2016; Wu & Wu, 2012). During the last two decades, the role of gut bacteria in health and disease has been at the centre of our attention. The role of dysbiosis (i.e. unbalanced bacterial composition in the gut) on autoimmune disorders and mental diseases such as autism, depression, and anxiety is under investigation (Pugliese et al., 2022). Studies indicate a link between Caesarean birth and diseases such as asthma, chronic inflammatory bowel disease, and diabetes, as the neonate will be infected with hospital bacteria instead of the mother's bacteria through the birth canal (Neu & Rushing, 2011). Antibiotic treatment early in life will skew the balance in bacterial composition and can therefore also be a link to autoimmune diseases (Schulfer & Blaser, 2015).

Modern technology has enabled us to understand the complexities of the microbial communities in a symbiotic relationship with human cells (Figure 13.2), yet our understanding of viral components is largely in its infancy. However, technology has shed light on the evolution of the human genome, genetic diseases and the development of gene therapies.

During COVID-19 pandemic millions of human lives were lost in addition to the social and economic costs (Cutler & Summers, 2020). We welcome the end of the pandemic, but the disease remains and is endemic. COVID-19

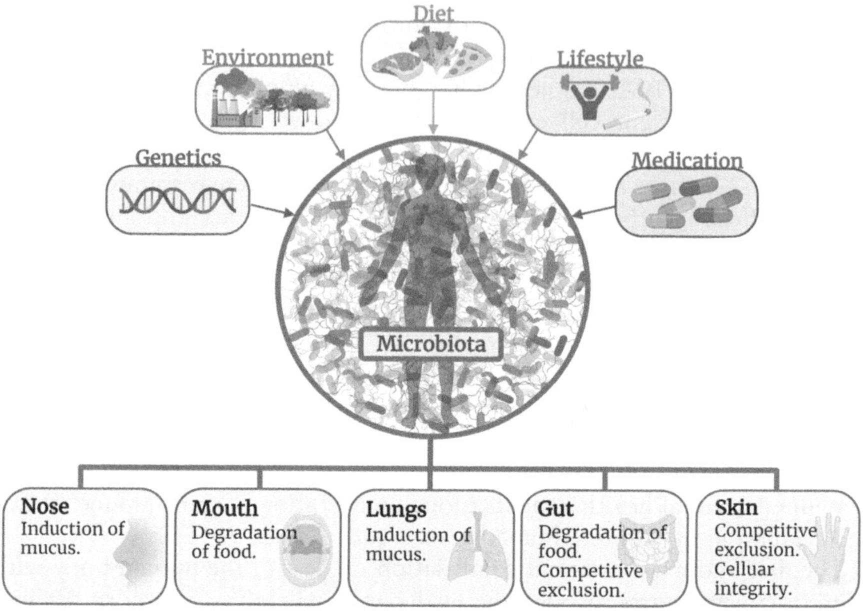

Figure 13.2 Schematic presentation of different factors affecting the human microbiota. Subsequently, the human microbiota affects human health by, e.g., inducing mucus production in the nose, lungs, and gut, thus protecting against pathogens, producing enzymes to degrade food in the mouth and gut, and providing homeostasis and competitive exclusion of pathogens in the gut and on the skin, as well as many other effects.

clearly changed human behaviour from socialisation to isolation. This occurred through public health guidelines from the authorities focusing on social distancing, wearing masks, intense hand sanitisation, working from home, shopping online, etc. However, exposure to a diversity of microorganisms through socialisation establishes a stronger and healthier microbiota in the host and strengthens the immune system. The first signs of this under-stimulation of the immune system are seen after two years of social distancing. As early as January 2022, when life was back to normal after two years of social distancing, many reports showed that people were more prone to becoming ill with, e.g., influenza or other common viral infections (https://www.weforum.org/agenda/2023/02/other-infections-rising-since-covid-pandemic/).

The interactions between human cells and the microorganisms colonising the human body are important to understand both during symbiotic relationship, but also when disease occurs. These interactions are important for understanding SARS-CoV-2 pathogenesis. The interactions are important for understanding SARS-CoV-2 pathogenesis in order to develop novel treatment and means of prevention in spreading the virus.

The effects of COVID-19 on our health and behaviour, and the future consequences for our health and lifestyle, are here discussed.

Gut microbiota in health and disease

Gut microbiota

The early history of microbiology starts in the 1670s, when the first microscope became available and scientist Robert Hooke observed strands of fungi among cells (Corliss, 2002). Subsequently, Anton Van Leeuwenhoek made observations of 'animalcules' such as protozoa, fungi, and bacteria. In the late 19th century, known as 'the golden age of microbiology', Louis Pasteur discovered penicillin and thereby the role of bacteria in health and disease (Corliss, 2002). However, working with viruses was more challenging. It required an electron microscope, which was not developed until the 1940s, after which viruses were discovered (Corliss, 2002).

The benefits of natural microbial compositions have been used to cure disease since the 4th century BC, as the first use of healthy donor faeces (faecal microbiota transplantation) as a therapeutic agent for food poisoning and diarrhoea was recorded in the *Chinese Handbook of Emergency Medicine* (Hong Ge) (Gaines & Alverdy, 2017). Kefir, which is a fermented probiotic drink, has been in use for thousands of years by people in the Caucasus mountains to improve digestion, lower blood pressure and cholesterol, prevent cancer, improve the immune system, and reduce asthma and allergies (Kim & Yi, 2020).

The role of bacteria in the gut in health and disease

The human gastrointestinal tract is one of the most complex organ systems of the human body, where a symbiotic relationship between associated microbiota and the host is essential. The gastrointestinal tract starts at the mouth and ends at the anus, having a total length of nine metres. Among the most vital residents of the human gut are bacteria. They play an essential role in human health and disease, as we cannot live without them, and they can cause disease, even death, in the host. There is still much to learn about gut bacteria, as we have only discovered the tip of the iceberg. Over 50% of gut bacteria are in fact not culturable, and therefore difficult to study (Corliss, 2002).

Bacteria interact with other bacteria and human cells by:

- Communicating with one another (bacteria-bacterial and bacteria-eukaryote) through hormone-like signals to modulate their gene expression, known as 'quorum sensing'.
- Modifying human cell-signal transduction.

The first time the human body is introduced to bacteria is through the birth canal, after which infants become exposed to bacteria through their mother's breast milk (Kim & Yi, 2020) and later on through factors such as water, food, and the surrounding environment. It is during the first years of life that the human immune response is shaped. Therefore, certain bacteria and macromolecules play a critical role in stimulating and training the immune system to behave in certain ways. Studies show that children raised in homes with pets are often free from asthma and allergies, while children living in inner cities or who grew up in excessively clean environments, develop hypersensitive immune systems that make them prone to asthma and allergies (Wood, 2014).

Diet is an important factor to form and modulate the human intestinal bacterial community. Studies show that a high daily intake of fast food, rich in digestible sugars, fats (beef, pork, corn, and margarines) is linked to overweight, a leaky gut, dysbiosis, and chronic diseases such as inflammatory bowel disease and diabetes (Burisch et al., 2014). However, a Mediterranean diet rich in non-digestible fibres, such as vegetables, wholewheat bread, fish, olive oil, fruits, and nuts (D'Souza et al., 2008), is linked to healthy gut bacteria (Mirsepasi-Lauridsen et al., 2019). Human gut bacteria ferment dietary carbohydrates and fibres to short-chain fatty acids (SCFAs). SCFAs, such as acetate propionate and butyrate, all have anti-inflammatory effects and inhibit bacterial overgrowth in the gut (Viladomiu et al., 2013). The rate of the SCFA produced depends on the richness of specific bacteria in the colon (Wolin, 1969). SCFAs serve as a major source of energy for colonic epithelial cells and are an inhibitor of proinflammatory cytokine expression in the intestinal mucosa. Less than 1% of the colon bacteria use their metabolic pathways to produce SCFA (Smith & Huggins, 1983; Smith & MacFarlane, 1998).

The symbiotic relationship of human and bacteria cells is based on humans coexisting with bacteria for potential mutual benefit, as bacteria use host food to cover their needs and produce metabolites, such as SCFAs, which are beneficial for human health (Wolin, 1969). When this chain is broken by, for instance, a wrong diet or increased usage of antibiotics early in life, it will promote an imbalance between the gut bacteria (dysbiosis). This will cause specific bacteria to overgrow and thereby change the gut environment to become optimal for them (Mirsepasi-Lauridsen, 2022). Dysbiosis is linked to a number of chronic diseases, such as inflammatory bowel disease, Alzheimer's disease, Parkinson's disease, cancer, obesity, heart diseas e, and chronic infections (Hou et al., 2022; van de Wouw, 2018).

Dysbiosis is also linked to SARS-CoV-2 pathogenesis, since SARS-CoV-2 uses angiotensin-converting enzyme 2 (ACE2) that attaches to the cells as an entry point, causing ACE2 malfunction (Figure 13.3) (Zhang et al., 2020b). ACE2 is an enzyme attached to the membrane of cells in the intestines, kidneys, testis, gall bladder, and heart, or it can be in a soluble form (Chen et al., 2020; Hikmet et al., 2020). Both soluble and membrane-bound ACE2 form an integral part of the renin-angiotensin-aldosterone system that exists to keep the body blood pressure in check. A malfunction of ACE2 expression

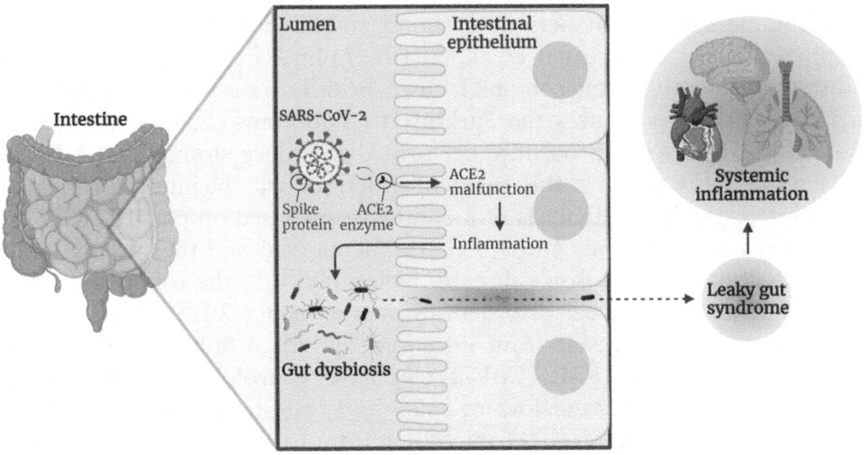

Figure 13.3 Effect of SARS-CoV-2 on gut dysbiosis by causing malfunction of the ACE2 enzyme.

in the gut can lead to increased gut permeability/leaky gut, followed by dysbiosis (Hashimoto et al., 2012). Therefore, ACE2 is a potential target molecule for SARS-CoV-2 disease treatment. Yet a healthy gut microbiota should be able to prevent disease in the gut from SARS-CoV-2.

Clinical studies indicate that a coinfection with SARS-CoV-2 changes the intestinal homeostasis and stimulates immune cells to overproduce cytokines causing severe inflammation. Studies indicate a significant reduction in intestinal bacterial diversity in SARS-CoV-2 patients with a relative abundance of opportunistic pathogens such as the genera of *Streptococcus*, *Rothia*, *Veillonella*, and *Actinomyces*, and decreased amounts of beneficial bacteria such as *Blautia*, *Romboutsia*, and *Bifidobacterium* (Gu et al., 2020). Increased prevalence of fungi such as *Aspergillus* spp., *Candida albicans*, and *Candida glabrata* was also reported in SARS-CoV-2 patients. However, 70% of the patients included in the study were treated with antibiotics, which promotes the prevalence of fungi in patients (Chen et al., 2020; Rouse & Sehrawat, 2010). In the past decade, the link between gut bacteria and the brain has been at the centre of attention (Hou et al., 2022). There is a growing body of evidence indicating that the gut bacteria exert a profound influence on key brain processes, which led to the development of the concept 'microbiota-gut-brain axis' (Erny et al., 2015; Wang et al., 2019). Gut bacteria can influence the central nervous system processes through the vagus nerve (Rhee et al., 2009), by modulating the immune system through tryptophan metabolism along with their ability to synthesise several neurotransmitters and by producing metabolites such as SCFAs that possess neuroactive properties (Fleming & Floch, 1986; Fung et al., 2020). SCFAs influence gut-brain communication and brain function directly and indirectly, e.g. by contributing to the biosynthesis of serotonin, and improving neuronal homeostasis and function. Serotonin is a chemical messenger that acts as a mood stabiliser and promotes healthy sleeping patterns (Szentirmai et al., 2019). Animal experiments show that transferring faecal/gut microbiota from a healthy mouse to a mouse with Parkinson's disease reduces the Parkinson's symptoms (Fung et al., 2020). Truncal vagotomy is a procedure performed to reduce stomach acid, by removing the vagus nerves of the stomach, which connect the intestines with the brain. Interestingly, an analysis of a cohort study based on patients who underwent truncal vagotomy showed that patients who had the surgery had a clear reduction in Parkinson's disease, which indicates the role of intestinal microbiota in neurological disorders (Svensson et al., 2015). Thus, neurological disorders can result from intestinal dysbiosis. Studies indicate that patients infected with SARS-CoV-2 can have neurological complications ranging from headache and loss of smell and taste to confusion, disabling strokes and other long-term chronic complications (Hamming et al., 2004; Iadecola et al., 2020).

The role of bacteriophages in symbiosis and dysbiosis

Bacteriophages are viruses that infect bacteria and play an essential role in many natural ecosystems. They outnumber bacteria by a factor of 10 and have a strong influence on bacterial diversity and population size (Riley, 2004). Bacteriophages are known to be immunogenic and have been used to access humoral immune functions, such as bacteriophages-based vaccines (Riley, 2004). They can modify gut bacteria communities by modulating immune agents or via steric competition for microbe-associated molecular patterns on bacterial surfaces (Hassan et al., 2021; Riley, 2004). Bacteriophages might play an essential role in gut bacteria dysbiosis by destabilising bacterial communities and by gene transfer and genome reorganisation within the bacteria population (Bohnsack et al. 1985; Norman et al., 2015). New bacteria carrying phages or already residing lysogenic bacteriophages can infect normal gut bacteria, causing the release of large amounts of phage proteins, which promote dysbiosis. However, environmental factors such as smoking are also known to trigger this process (Riley, 2004). Bacteriophages can play a role in bacterial pathogenesis, e.g. toxin genes of *Streptococcus pyogenes* strains that cause scarlet fever are carried by a temperate bacteriophage (Riley, 2004).

Role of human viruses in the gut

Virus in Latin means poison and viruses are one of the most abundant of all evolutionary entities (Lasso et al., 2019). Eight percent of the human genome is a sequence that is related to retroviruses, and there are >1000 types of viruses that are estimated to infect humans (Moelling & Broecker, 2019). Viral infections attack a wide range of tissues and organs such as the upper respiratory tract and lungs (e.g. the influenza virus and coronavirus) (Dimmock et al., 2016), the colon (e.g. the rotavirus), the liver (e.g. the hepatitis B virus) (Lang et al., 2006), the spinal cord (e.g. the polio virus) (Lang et al., 2006), vascular endothelial cells (e.g. Ebola) (Kaner & Schaack, 2016), and white blood cells (e.g. HIV) (Dimmock et al., 2016).

When viruses are exposed to mucosal surfaces such as in the intestine, they have three broad lines of defence to overcome: the mucus layer, nonspecific immunity known as the innate immune defence, and the adaptive immune defence based on specialised systemic cells and processes (Lang et al., 2006). Antiviral mechanisms also enhance mucosal barrier function (Lang et al., 2006), secretion of antiviral antimicrobial peptides (Lang et al., 2006), bacteriocins (Su et al., 2013), inhibition of viral attachment to host cells and modulation of antiviral innate and adaptive leucocyte function (Su et al., 2013). Bacteriocins are driven by probiotic/beneficial bacteria that display antiviral activity before viruses enter human cells. An example of this is duramycin which is produced by streptomycetes and prevents the Zika virus from entering human cells by blocking its co-receptor (Su et al., 2013).

Viral infections have been causing pandemics for centuries and have cost millions of human lives. Smallpox caused by the variola virus resulted in 300–500 million deaths in the 20th century. HIV infected 79.3 million people and has killed 47.8 million to date and SARS-CoV-2, since late 2019, has infected >679 million and killed >6.88 million to date (https://www.who.int). Coronavirus infects the upper airways and the lungs, causing fever, cough, dyspnoea, anosmia, and fatigue (Su et al., 2013) in addition to systemic presentations including cardiovascular, haematological, renal, neurological, dermatological, and gastrointestinal manifestations (Gupta et al., 2020). However, it is unknown whether these systemic presentations are caused directly by SARS-CoV-2 or indirectly by the excessive release of cytokines, by thromboembolic effects impairing microcirculation or by a combination of all these complications (Braun et al., 2020; Escher et al., 2020; Meinhardt et al., 2021).

Studies show that the prevalence of SARS-CoV-2 RNA in stool samples from positive cases was 48.1% and of those 70.3% remained positive for viral RNA in the stools, even when respiratory specimens were tested negative (Cheung et al., 2020). SARS-CoV-2 was also found in the biopsies from intestinal tissues of individuals who were infected with SARS-CoV-2 (Lin et al., 2020b). SARS-CoV-2 has been shown to replicate in the microvilli-colonic cell line C2BBe1 (Escher et al., 2020) and also within cells of human small intestinal organoids derived from primary human small intestinal epithelial stem cells. SARS-CoV-2 uses ACE2 as an entry receptor, which is highly expressed on differentiated enterocytes. ACE2 regulates innate immunity and microbial ecology in the intestine and a deficiency of ACE2 causes epithelial damage followed by intestinal inflammation (Hashimoto et al., 2012). Clinical studies show that patients infected with SARS-CoV-2 have a high incidence of comorbidities such as hypertension, diabetes mellitus, coronary heart disease, and cerebrovascular disease, which are all linked to ACE2 enzyme malfunction (Figure 13.3) (Zhang et al., 2020).

Studies show that symptoms of SARS-CoV-2 can persist for months, caused by damage to the lungs, heart, and brain. Some of the symptoms are fatigue, difficulty breathing, coughing, problems with memory, concentration or sleeping, fast heartbeat, depression or anxiety, dizziness when standing, with worsened symptoms after physical or mental activities. Some experience multisystem inflammatory syndromes after infection with SARS-CoV-2, where some organs and tissues become severely inflamed. Blood clots were also reported following SARS-CoV-2 infection, which affected the lungs, legs, liver, and kidneys (Lopez-Leon et al., 2021). SARS-CoV-2 infected patients were seen to have an increased the prevalence of respiratory viruses, such as non-SARS-CoV-2 coronaviruses, entero/rhinoviruses and respiratory syncytial viruses (Lin et al., 2020b). Since SARS-CoV-2 infection causes damage to the epithelium through malfunction of ACE2, resulting in an increase of viral coinfections (Lin et al., 2020a). Viruses can also cause immune system disorders thus increase the likelihood of infection by other viruses (Rouse & Sehrawat, 2010). The long-term effects of SARS-CoV-2 on infected people are still unknown, but research is ongoing. Yet one thing is certain, namely that COVID-19 affects our present behaviour in terms of more social distancing, and increased hygiene of hands, utensils, surfaces, and food packaging. However, as mentioned previously, the human immune defence needs environmental microbiota and allergens as well as social contact, to introduce the immune system to new microbiota, thereby enabling the stimulation and training of the immune system. SARS-CoV-2 changed human behaviour and living standards towards living in excessively clean environments with potential future consequences in the form of a hypersensitive immune system. These and other aspects will be discussed in the next section.

What have we learned from past pandemics?

Lessons from past pandemics

Before the 1940s, bacterial infections were responsible for the deaths of millions of people throughout history, e.g. the pandemics of tuberculosis (Hamming et al., 2004), diphtheria (Opinel & Gachelin, 2011), syphilis (Aminov, 2010), typhus, and bubonic plague. The bubonic plague, also known as the 'Black Death', was caused by the bacterium *Yersinia pestis* and killed 75 million people at its peak in the 14th century, equal to one-third of the world population at that time (Aminov, 2010). Tuberculosis at its peak in the 19th century was responsible for the death of one billion people, which makes it the second biggest global killer in history after malaria (Barberis et al., 2017). These diseases are scarce in the modern world, but it would be foolish to forget the importance of antibiotics and vaccines, which partly eradicated these diseases. Modern medicine has fought an impressive battle against these pathogenic bacteria and viruses, but the threat has not been completely erased, especially considering the current health threats sweeping the world including the rise of multi-antibiotic-resistant organisms (Shams et al., 2016).

Challenges for gut microbiota when using antibiotics

Antibiotics in the form of medical plant extracts were used over 2000 years ago by the ancient Egyptians and Greeks. It was not until 1928, when Alexander Fleming noticed that the green mould, *Penicillium rubens*, killed or prevented the growth of bacteria, that the production of antibiotics commenced (Forrest, 1982). The period from the 1950s to the 1980s is known as the 'golden age' of antibiotic discovery. In this period, countless new classes of antibiotics were discovered and used to treat incurable diseases, such as tuberculosis and syphilis (Forrest, 1982; Tan & Tatsumura, 2015). Then began the massive production of synthetic antibiotic chemotherapeutics to combat pathogenic bacteria. With increased usage of antibiotic chemotherapy, the phenomenon of resistance was discovered, consisting of bacterial strains with physiologically or genetically enhanced capacity to survive antibiotics. The most frequently used antibiotics, such as penicillin and erythromycin, became less effective with time, due to the increased resistance of many bacterial strains (Innes et al. 2020).

As antibiotic-resistant bacteria ('superbugs') rapidly increased and promoted dysbiosis in the gut, the World Health Organization Advisory Group implemented surveillance of antimicrobial resistance, and recommended reducing the usage of medically important antimicrobials in livestock for, e.g., growth promotion and disease prevention (Innes et al., 2020).

Antimicrobial resistance threatens humankind and can lead to epidemics if preventative actions are not taken. It leads to longer hospitalisation, higher medical costs, and increased mortality (WHO, 2014). Antibiotic therapy in humans has a great impact on gut bacteria, as it alters the bacterial count in the gut, causing irritation of the gut mucosa follow by diarrhoea and reduced ability to digest food (Shams et al., 2016). Antibiotic therapy can change the levels of microbiota in the gut (dysbiosis) and allow pathogenic bacteria such as *C. difficile* to overgrow (Shams et al., 2016). When a patient is treated with antibiotics over a long period, it can promote antibiotic-resistant bacteria, which invade the human gut, causing illnesses that are difficult to treat with antibiotics (Braun et al., 2020).

Since SARS-CoV-2 was reported to overlap or be followed by bacterial infection, antibiotic therapy in a SARS-CoV-2-infected patient was suggested as a basic principle of treatment (Bassetti et al., 2020; Langford, 2021). According to the published data, patients with viral pneumonia and bacterial or fungal coinfection have a higher mortality rate if not treated appropriately (Bengoechea & Bamford, 2020). Despite the strong recommendation for surveillance of antimicrobial resistance to reduce the use of antimicrobial therapy, in the early phase of the COVID-19 pandemic more than 75% of hospitalised SARS-CoV-2 infected patients received antibiotic therapy, while only 8% of the patients were confirmed as having bacterial coinfection (Mohamad et al., 2022; Yang et al., 2020b). During the pandemic, antibiotic prescriptions were extensive and excessive (Li et al., 2020), while only 1–10% of the patients were reported as having SARS-CoV-2 coinfection (Huang et al., 2020).

With this knowledge, we need to be prepared for increased occurrence of multidrug-resistant bacteria in the future, and increased prevalence of gut dysbiosis in SARS-CoV-2 infected patients treated with antibiotics. Most clinicians justified the use of antibiotics in the early stages of the COVID-19 pandemic, based on clinical assessment. However, a study from Malaysia showed that reduced use of antibiotics and increased use of antiviral and anti-malarial agents was effective to promote recovery in SARS-CoV-2 infected patients (Mohamad et al., 2022).

The COVID-19 pandemic affected human gut microbiota in many ways such as:

- By stress-induced leaky gut/dysbiosis, leading to immune deficiencies and other chronic disorders
- By malfunction of ACE2 enzyme expression on the microvilli colonic cells, caused by SARS-CoV-2 infection, leading to dysbiosis followed by anxiety and depression (Sørensen et al., 2022)

Challenges with vaccine development during pandemics

Vaccination originates from a centuries-old practice called inoculation, which took place in the Middle East and China for hundreds of years before it made its way to Europe during the 18th century. The method was based on inserting a small amount of preserved bacteria under the skin of a healthy person, to give that person a controlled dose of the disease leading to immunisation, Edward Jenner's presented his systematic findings at the Royal Society of London in 1796 detailing his success in preventing smallpox by inoculation with live infectious material from the pustules or scabs of people infected with cowpox. The process induced cowpox, a mild viral disease that conferred immunity to smallpox. Jenner called the cowpox material 'vaccine' (from *vacca*, the Latin for cow) and the process vaccination. Later, better vaccine production techniques were discovered, after which the British government in 1853 made vaccination mandatory and free of charge (Wolfe & Sharp, 2002).

Vaccine development is a long, complex process and may take 10–15 years, with a combination of public and private involvement (Wolfe & Sharp, 2002). In the late 19th century, several vaccines for humans were developed, such as those against smallpox, rabies, and the plague. However, no regulation of vaccine production existed at that time. Not until 1902 did the US congress pass an act to regulate the sale of viruses, serums, toxins, and analogous products, later referred to as the Biologics Control Act, to control the quality of drugs (Wolfe & Sharp, 2002). This act required hygienic laboratories for production and different stages of vaccine development and testing, in which over 10 000 participants were involved (Wolfe & Sharp, 2002).

Realising the magnitude of the COVID-19 pandemic and the necessity for very prompt action, researchers combined previous knowledge and in early 2020, the FDA announced approval of three SARS-CoV-2 vaccine candidates that had been selected for testing in humans. In January 2021, several countries initiated a SARS-CoV-2 vaccination programme for the more vulnerable population.

What to do during future pandemics

The COVID-19 pandemic and the development of vaccines in such a short time taught us to use previous knowledge from other fields and novel technologies to combat infectious threats. Collaboration across disciplines is essential for success. In addition, fast processing by the authorities of legal ethical approvals for vaccine testing and accelerating vaccine production brought COVID-19 under control relatively quickly.

Fast actions on the pandemic from the governments such as social distancing, focusing on hand sanitation, and mask wearing in public spaces were implemented in all countries.

The actions of governments and the World Health Organization during COVID-19 were based on knowledge gained from history. However, novel disease outbreaks of the scale of SARS-CoV-2 are predicted to become more likely in the future, but thanks to our experience in managing this pandemic, we are better equipped to manage future outbreaks. The key lessons from the COVID-19 pandemic will help to improve trust in science, inspire positive health behaviour and prevent spreading of diseases as they emerge.

References

Abdolmaleki, G., Taheri, M. A., Paridehpour, S., Mohammadi, N. M., Tabatabaei, Y. A., Mousavi, T., & Amin, M. (2022). A comparison between SARS-CoV-1 and SARS-CoV2: An update on current COVID-19 vaccines. *DARU: Journal of Faculty of Pharmacy, Tehran University of Medical Sciences*, *30*(2), 379–406. Available at: 10.1007/s40199-022-00446-8.

Aminov, R. I. (2010). A brief history of the antibiotic era: Lessons learned and challenges for the future. *Frontiers in Microbiology*, *1*, 1–7.

Barberis, I., Bragazzi, N. L., Galluzzo, L., & Martini, M. (2017). The history of tuberculosis: From the first historical records to the isolation of Koch's bacillus. *Journal of Preventive Medicine and Hygiene*, *58*(1), 9–12.

Bassetti, M., Giacobbe, D. R., Aliberti, S., Barisione, E., Centanni, S., De Rosa, F. G., Di Marco, F., Gori, A., Granata, G., Mikulska, M., Petrosillo, N., Richeldi, L., Santus, P., Tascini, C., Vena, A., Viale, P., & Blasi, F. (2020). Balancing evidence and frontline experience in the early phases of the COVID-19 pandemic: Current position of the Italian Society of Antiinfective Therapy (SITA) and the Italian Society of Pulmonology (SIP). *Clinical Microbiology and Infection*, *26*(7), 880–894.

Beaven, S. W. (2004). Biomarkers in inflammatory bowel disease. *Current Opinion in Gastroenterology*, *20*(4), 318–327. Available at: http://journals.lww.com/co-gastroenterology/Abstract/2004/07000/Biomarkers_in_inflammatory_bowel_disease.4.aspx%5Cnpapers2://publication/uuid/0937EC3F-23BC-4024-82ED-E675499073B5.

Bengoechea, J. A., & Bamford, C. G. G. (2020). SARS-CoV-2, bacterial co-infections, and AMR: The deadly trio in COVID-19? *EMBO Molecular Medicine*, *12*(7), 10–13.

Bohnsack, J., Ochs, H. D., Wedgwood, R. J., & Heller, S. R. (1985). Antibody to bacteriophage phi X 174 synthesized by cultured human peripheral blood lymphocytes. *Clinical and Experimental Immunology*, *59*(3), 673–678.

Burisch, J., Pedersen, N., Cukovic-Cavka, S., Turk, N., Kaimakliotis, I., Duricova, D., Bortlik, M., Shonová, O., Vind, I., Avnstrøm, S., Thorsgaard, N., Krabbe, S., Andersen, V., Dahlerup, J. F., Kjeldsen, J., Salupere, R., Olsen, J., Nielsen, K. R., Manninen, P., & Munkholm, P. (2014). Environmental factors in a population-based inception cohort of inflammatory bowel disease patients in Europe – An ECCO-EpiCom study. *Journal of Crohn's and Colitis*, *8*(7), 607–616.

Braun, F., Lutgehetmann, M., Pfefferle, S., Wong, M. N., Carsten, A., Lindenmeyer, M. T., Nörz, D., Heinrich, F., Meissner, K., Wichmann, D., Kluge, S., Gross, O., Pueschel, K., Schröder, A. S., Edler, C., Aepfelbacher, M., Puelles, V. G., & Huber, T. B. (2020). SARS-CoV-2 renal tropism associates with acute kidney injury. *The Lancet*, *396*, 597–598.

Chen, N., Zhou, M., Dong, X., Qu, J., Gong, F., Han, Y., Qiu, Y., Wang, J., Liu, Y., Wei, Y., Xia, J., Yu, T., Zhang, X., & Zhang, L. (2020). Epidemiological and clinical characteristics of 99 cases of 2019 novel coronavirus pneumonia in Wuhan, China: A descriptive study. *The Lancet*, *395*(10223), 507–513.

Cheung, K. S., Hung, I. F. N., Chan, P. P. Y., Lung, K. C., Tso, E., Liu, R., Ng, Y. Y., Chu, M. Y., Chung, T. W. H., Tam, A. R., Yip, C. C. Y., Leung, K.-H., Fung, A. Y.-F., Zhang, R. R., Lin, Y., Cheng, H. M., Zhang, A. J. X., To, K. K. W., Chan, K.-H., ...Leung, W. K. (2020). Gastrointestinal manifestations of SARS-CoV-2 infection and virus load in fecal samples from a Hong Kong cohort: Systematic review and meta-analysis. *Gastroenterology*, *159*(1), 81–95.

Corliss, J. O. (2002). A salute to Antony van Leeuwenhoek of Delft, most versatile 17th century founding father of protistology. *Protist*, *153*(2), 177–190.

Cutler, D. M., & Summers, L. H. (2020). The COVID-19 pandemic and the $16 trillion virus. *JAMA*, *324*(15), 1495–1496.

Dimmock, N. J., Easton, A. J., & Leppard, K. N. (2016). *Introduction to modern virology* (7th ed.). John Wiley & Sons.

D'Souza, S., Levy, E., Mack, D., Israel, D., Lambrette, P., Ghadirian, P., Morgan, K., Seidman, E. G., & Amre, D. K. (2008). Dietary patterns and risk for Crohn's disease in children. *Inflammatory Bowel Diseases*, *14*(3), 367–373.

Ellwanger, J. H., & Chies, J. A. B. (2021). Zoonotic spillover: Understanding basic aspects for better prevention. *Genetics and Molecular Biology*, *44*(1), 1–18.

Erny, D., De Angelis, A. L. H., Jaitin, D., Wieghofer, P., Staszewski, O., David, E., et al. (2015) Host microbiota constantly control maturation and function of microglia in the CNS. *Nature Neuroscience*, *18*, 965–977. doi: 10.1038/nn.4030 7.

Escher, F., Pietsch, H., Aleshcheva, G., Bock, T., Baumeier, C., Elsaesser, A., Wenzel, P., Hamm, C., Westenfeld, R., Schultheiss, M., Gross, U., Morawietz, L., & Schultheiss, H.-P. (2020). Detection of viral SARS-CoV-2 genomes and histopathological changes in endomyocardial biopsies. *ESC Heart Failure*, *7*(5), 2440–2447.

Fekadu, G., Bekele, F., Tolossa, T., Fetensa, G., Turi, E., Getachew, M., Abdisa, E., Assefa, L., Afeta, M., Demisew, W., Dugassa, D., Diriba, D. C., & Labata, B. G. (2021). Impact of COVID-19 pandemic on chronic diseases care follow-up and current perspectives in low resource settings: A narrative review. *International Journal of Physiology, Pathophysiology and Pharmacology*, *13*(3), 86–93. Available at: http://www.ncbi.nlm.nih.gov/pubmed/34336132%0Ahttp://www.pubmedcentral.nih.gov/articlerender.fcgi?artid=PMC8310882.

Fleming, L. L., & Floch, M. H. (1986). Digestion and absorption of fiber carbohydrate in the colon. *The American Journal of Gastroenterology*, *81*(7), 507–511.

Forrest, R. D. (1982). Early history of wound treatment. *Journal of the Royal Society of Medicine*, *75*, 198–205.

Fung, T. C., Olson, C. A., & Hsiao, E. Y. (2020). Interactions between the microbiota, immune and nervous systems in health and disease. *Nature Neuroscience*, *20*(2), 145–155.

Gaines, S., & Alverdy, J. C. (2017). Fecal microbiota transplantation to treat sepsis of unclear etiology. *Critical Care Medicine*, *45*, 1106–1107.

Gardner, C. L., & Ryman, K. D. (2010). Yellow fever: A reemerging threat. *Clinics in Laboratory Medicine*, *30*, 237–260.

Gu, S., Chen, Y., Wu, Z., Chen, Y., Hainv, G., Lv, L., Guo, F., Zhang, X., Luo, R., Huang, C., Lu, H., Zheng, B., Zhang, J., Yan, R., Huan, Z., Jiang, H., Xu, Q., Guo, J., Gong, Y., & Li, L. (2020). Alterations of the gut microbiota in patients with COVID-19 or H1N1 influenza. *Clinical Infectious Diseases*, *71*(10), 2669–2678.

Gupta, A., Madhavan, M. V., Sehgal, K., Nair, N., Mahajan, S., Sehrawat, T. S., Bikdeli, B., Ahluwalia, N., Ausiello, J. C., Wan, E. Y., Freedberg, D. E., Kirtane, A. J., Parikh, S. A., Maurer, M. S., Nordvig, A. S., Accili, D., Bathon, J. M., Mohan, S., Bauer, K. A., ...Landry, D. W. (2020). Extrapulmonary manifestations of COVID-19. *Nature Medicine*, *26*(7), 1017–1032. Available at: 10.1038/s41591-020-0968-3.

Hamming, I., Timens, W., Bulthuis, M. L. C., Lely, A. T., Navis, G. J., & van Goor, H. (2004). Tissue distribution of ACE2 protein, the functional receptor for SARS coronavirus. A first step in understanding SARS pathogenesis. *The Journal of Pathology*, *203*(2), 631–637.

Hashimoto, T., Perlot, T., Rehman, A., Trichereau, J., Ishiguro, H., Paolino, M., Sigl, V., Hanada, T., Hanada, R., Lipinski, S., Wild, B., Camargo, S. M. R., Singer, D., Richter, A., Kuba, K., Fukamizu, A., Schreiber, S., Clevers, H., Verrey, F., & Penninger, J. M. (2012). ACE2 links amino acid malnutrition to microbial ecology and intestinal inflammation. *Nature*, *487*(7408), 4–10.

Hassan, A. Y., Lin, J. T., Ricker, N., & Anany, H. (2021). The age of phage: Friend or foe in the new dawn of therapeutic and biocontrol applications? *Pharmaceuticals (Basel)*, *14*(3), 1–35.

Hikmet, F., Méar, L., Edvinsson, Å., Micke, P., Uhlén, M., & Lindskog, C. (2020). The protein expression profile of ACE2 in human tissues. *Molecular Systems Biology*, *16*(7), 1–16.

Hou, K., Wu, Z.-X., Chen, X.-Y., Wang, J.-Q., Zhang, D., Xiao, C., Zhu, D., Koya, J. B., Wei, L., Li, J., & Chen, Z.-S. (2022). Microbiota in health and diseases. *Signal Transduction and Targeted Therapy*, *7*(1), 135.

Huang, C., Wang, Y., Li, X., Ren, L., Zhao, J., Hu, Y., Zhang, L., Fan, G., Xu, J., Gu, X., Cheng, Z., Yu, T., Xia, J., Wei, Y., Wu, W., Xie, X., Yin, W., Li, H., Liu, M., & Cao, B. (2020). Clinical features of patients infected with 2019 novel coronavirus in Wuhan, China. *Lancet*, *395*(10223), 497–506.

Iadecola, C., Anrather, J., & Kamel, H. (2020). Effects of COVID-19 on the nervous system. *Cell*, *183*(1), 16–27.

Innes, G. K., Randad, P. R., Korinek, A., Davis, M. F., Price, L. B., So, A. D., & Heaney, C. D. (2020). External societal costs of antimicrobial resistance in humans attributable to antimicrobial use in livestock. *Annual Review of Public Health*, *41*, 141–157.

Kaner, J., & Schaack, S. (2016). Understanding Ebola: The 2014 epidemic. *Global Health*, *12*(1), 1–7. Available at: 10.1186/s12992-016-0194-4.

Kim, S. Y., & Yi, D. Y. (2020). Components of human breast milk: From macronutrient to microbiome and microRNA. *Clinical and Experimental Pediatrics*, *63*(8), 301–309.

Lang, C. A., Conrad, S., Garrett, L., Battistutta, D., Cooksley, W. G. E., Dunne, M. P., & Macdonald, G. A. (2006). Symptom prevalence and clustering of symptoms in people living with chronic hepatitis C infection. *Journal of Pain and Symptom Management*, *31*(4), 335–344.

Langford, B. J., So, M., Raybardhan, S., Leung, V., Soucy, J.-P. R., Westwood, D., Daneman, N., & MacFadden, D. R. (2021). Antibiotic prescribing in patients with COVID-19: Rapid review and meta-analysis. *Clinical Microbiology and Infection*, *27*(4), 520–531.

Lasso, G., Mayer, S. V., Winkelmann, E. R., Chu, T., Elliot, O., Patino-Galindo, J. A., et al. (2019). A Structure-informed atlas of human-virus interactions. *Cell*, *178*(1526–1541), e16. doi: 10.1016/j.cell.2019.08.005.

Li, Y., Ren, B., Peng, X., Hu, T., Li, J., Gong, T., Tang, B., Xu, X., & Zhou, X. (2020). Saliva is a non-negligible factor in the spread of COVID-19. *Molecular Oral Microbiology*, *35*(4), 141–145.

Lin, L., Jiang, X., Zhang, Z., Huang, S., Zhang, Z., Fang, Z., Gu, Z., Gao, L., Shi, H., Mai, L., Liu, Y., Lin, X., Lai, R., Yan, Z., Li, X., & Shan, H. (2020a). Gastrointestinal symptoms of 95 cases with SARS-CoV-2 infection. *Gut*, *69*(6), 997–1001.

Lin, D., Liu, L., Zhang, M., Hu, Y., Yang, Q., Guo, J., Guo, Y., Dai, Y., Xu, Y., Cai, Y., Chen, X., Zhang, Z., & Huang, K. (2020b). Co-infections of SARS-CoV-2 with multiple common respiratory pathogens in infected patients. *Science China Life Sciences*, *63*(4), 606–609.

Lopez-Leon, S., Wegman-Ostrosky, T., Perelman, C., Sepulveda, R., Rebolledo, P. A., Cuapio, A., & Villapol, S. (2021). More than 50 long-term effects of COVID-19: A systematic review and meta-analysis. *Scientific Reports 11*, 1–12. Available at: 10.1038/s41598-021-95565-8.

Meinhardt, J., Radke, J., Dittmayer, C., Franz, J., Thomas, C., Mothes, R., Laue, M., Schneider, J., Brünink, S., Greuel, S., Lehmann, M., Hassan, O., Aschman, T., Schumann, E., Chua, R. L., Conrad, C., Eils, R., Stenzel, W., Windgassen, M., ... Heppner, F. L. (2021). Olfactory transmucosal SARS-CoV-2 invasion as a port of central nervous system entry in individuals with COVID-19. *Nature Neuroscience*, *24*(2), 168–175. Available at: 10.1038/s41593-020-00758-5.

Mirsepasi-Lauridsen, H. C. (2022). Therapy used to promote disease remission targeting gut dysbiosis, in UC patients with active disease. *Journal of Clinical Medicine*, *11*(24), 7472.

Mirsepasi-Lauridsen, H. C., Vallance, B. A., Krogfelt, K. A., & Petersen, A. M. (2019). *Escherichia coli* pathobionts associated with inflammatory bowel disease. *Clinical Microbiology Reviews*, *32*(2), 1–16.

Moelling, K., & Broecker, F. (2019). Viruses and evolution – Viruses first? A personal perspective. *Frontiers in Microbiology*, *10*, 1–13.

Mohamad, I.-N., Wong, C. K.-W., Chew, C.-C., Leong, E.-L., Lee, B.-H., Moh, C.-K., Chenasammy, K., Lim, S. C.-L., & Ker, H.-B. (2022). The landscape of antibiotic usage among COVID-19 patients in the early phase of pandemic: A Malaysian national perspective. *Journal of Pharmaceutical Policy and Practice*, *15*(1), 4. Available at: 10.1186/s40545-022-00404-4.

Mueller, N. T., Bakacs, E., Combellick, J., Grigoryan, Z., & Dominguez-Bello, M. G. (2015). The infant microbiome development: Mom matters. *Trends in Molecular Medicine*, *21*(2), 109–117.

Neu, J., & Rushing, J. (2011). Cesarean versus vaginal delivery: Long-term infant outcomes and the hygiene hypothesis. *Clinics in Perinatology*, *38*(2), 321–331.

Norman, J. M., Handley, S. A., Baldridge, M. T., Droit, L., Liu, C. Y., Keller, B. C., et al. (2015). Disease-specific alterations in the enteric virome in inflammatory bowel disease. *Cell*, *160*, 447–460. doi: 10.1016/j.cell.2015.01.002.

Opinel, A., & Gachelin, G. (2011). French 19th century contributions to the development of treatments for diphtheria. *Journal of the Royal Society of Medicine*, *104*(4), 173–178.

Pugliese, D., Privitera, G., Fiorani, M., Parisio, L., Calvez, V., Papa, A., Gasbarrini, A., & Armuzzi, A. (2022). Targeting IL12/23 in ulcerative colitis: Update on the role of ustekinumab. *Therapeutic Advances in Gastroenterology*, *15*, 1–17.

Rhee, S. H., Pothoulakis, C., & Mayer, E. A. (2009). Principles and clinical implications of the brain-gut-enteric microbiota axis. *Nature Reviews Gastroenterology & Hepatology*, 6, 306–314. doi: 10.1038/nrgastro.2009.35.

Riley, P. A. (2004). Bacteriophages in autoimmune disease and other inflammatory conditions. *Medical Hypotheses*, *62*(4), 493–498. Available at: 10.1080/19490976.2022.2113717.

Rouse, B. T., & Sehrawat, S. (2010). Immunity and immunopathology to viruses: What decides the outcome? *Nature Reviews, Immunology*, *10*(7), 514–526. Available at: 10.1038/nri2802.36.

Schulfer, A., & Blaser, M. J. (2015). Risks of antibiotic exposures early in life on the developing microbiome. *PLoS Pathogens*, *11*(7), 1–6.

Sender, R., Fuchs, S., & Milo, R. (2016). Revised estimates for the number of human and bacteria cells in the body. *PLoS Biology*, *14*(8), 1–14.

Shams, A. M., Rose, L. J., Edwards, J. R., Cali, S., Harris, A. D., Jacob, J. T., LaFae, A., Pineles, L. L., Thom, K. A., McDonald, L. C., Arduino, M. J., & Noble-Wang, J. A. (2016). Assessment of the overall and multidrug-resistant organism bioburden on environmental surfaces in healthcare facilities. *Infection Control and Hospital Epidemiology*, *37*(12), 1426–1432.

Smith, E. A., & MacFarlane, G. T. (1998). Enumeration of amino acid fermenting bacteria in the human large intestine: Effects of pH and starch on peptide metabolism and dissimilation of amino acids. *FEMS Microbiology Ecology*, *25*(4), 355–368.

Smith, H. W., & Huggins, M. B. (1983). Effectiveness of phages in treating experimental *E. coli* diarrhoea in calves, piglets and lambs. *Journal of General Microbiology*, *129*, 2659–2675.

Sørensen, C. A., Clemmensen, A., Sparrewath, C., Tetens, M. M., & Krogfelt, K. A. (2022). Children naturally evading COVID-19 – Why children differ from adults. *COVID*, *2*(3), 369–378.

Su, Y., Zhang, B., & Su, L. (2013). CD4 detected from Lactobacillus helps understand the interaction between Lactobacillus and HIV. *Microbiological Research*, *168*(5), 273–277. Available at: 10.1016/j.micres.2012.12.004.

Svensson, E., Horváth-Puhó, E., Thomsen, R. W., Djurhuus, J. C., Pedersen, L., Borghammer, P., & Sørensen, H. T. (2015). Vagotomy and subsequent risk of Parkinson's disease. *Annals of Neurology*, *78*(4), 522–529.

Szentirmai, É., Millican, N. S., Massie, A. R., & Kapás, L. (2019). Butyrate, a metabolite of intestinal bacteria, enhances sleep. *Scientific Reports*, *9*(1), 7035.

Tan, S. Y., & Tatsumura, Y. (2015). Alexander Fleming (1881–1955): Discoverer of penicillin. *Singapore Medical Journal*, *56*(7), 366–367.

van de Wouw, M., Boehme, M., Lyte, J. M., Wiley, N., Strain, C., O'Sullivan, O., Clarke, G., Stanton, C., Dinan, T. G., & Cryan, J. F. (2018). Short-chain fatty acids: Microbial metabolites that alleviate stress-induced brain-gut axis alterations. *The Journal of Physiology*, *596*(20), 4923–4944.

Viladomiu, M., Hontecillas, R., Yuan, L., Lu, P., & Bassaganya-Riera, J. (2013). Nutritional protective mechanisms against gut inflammation. *The Journal of Nutritional Biochemistry*, *24*(6), 929–939.

Villarreal, L. P. (2005). *Viruses and the evolution of life*. ASM Press.

Wang, X., Sun, G., Feng, T., Zhang, J., Huang, X., Wang, T., Xie, Z., Chu, X., Yang, J., Wang, H., Chang, S., Gong, Y., Ruan, L., Zhang, G., Yan, S., Lian, W., Du, C., Yang, D., Zhang, Q., & Geng, M. (2019). Sodium oligomannate therapeutically remodels gut microbiota and suppresses gut bacterial amino acids-shaped neuroinflammation to inhibit Alzheimer's disease progression. *Cell Research*, *29*(10), 787–803. Available at: 10.1038/s41422-019-0216-x.40.

WHO. (2014). *Antimicrobial resistance, global report on surveillance*. World Health Organization. https://apps.who.int/iris/bitstream/handle/10665/112647/WHO_HSE_PED_AIP_2014.2_eng.pdf.

Wolfe, R. M., & Sharp, L. K. (2002). Anti-vaccinationists past and present. *British Medical Journal*, *325*(7361), 430–432.

Wolin, M. J. (1969). Volatile fatty acids and the inhibition of *Escherichia coli* growth by rumen fluid. *Applied Microbiology*, *17*(1), 83–87. Available at: http://eutils.ncbi.nlm.nih.gov/entrez/eutils/elink.fcgi?dbfrom=pubmed&id=4886864&retmode=ref&cmd=prlinks%5Cnpapers2://publication/uuid/36ADF05C-A39C-4FF4-97A0-135C60D87998.

Wood, R. A. (2014). *Pediatric allergy: An issue of immunology and allergy clinics of North America*. Elsevier.

Wu, H. J., & Wu, E. (2012). The role of gut microbiota in immune homeostasis and autoimmunity. *Gut Microbes*, *3*(1), 4–14.

Yang, Y., Peng, F., Wang, R., Yange, M., Guan, K., Jiang, T., Xu, G., Sun, J., & Chang, C. (2020a). The deadly coronaviruses: The 2003 SARS pandemic and the 2020 novel coronavirus epidemic in China. *Journal of Autoimmunity*, *109*, 102434. Available at: 10.1016/j.jaut.2020.102434.

Yang, X., Yu, Y., Xu, J., Shu, H., Xia, J., Liu, H., Wu, Y., Zhang, L., Yu, Z., Fang, M., Yu, T., Wang, Y., Pan, S., Zou, X., Yuan, S., & Shang, Y. (2020b). Clinical course and outcomes of critically ill patients with SARS-CoV-2 pneumonia in Wuhan, China: A single-centered, retrospective, observational study. *The Lancet Respiratory Medicine*, *8*(5), 475–481. Available at: 10.1016/S2213-2600(20)30079-5.

Zhang, Q., Zhang, H., Gao, J., Huang, K., Yang, Y., Hui, X., He, X., Li, C., Gong, W., Zhang, Y., Zhao, Y., Peng, C., Gao, X., Chen, H., Zou, Z., Shi, Z.-L., & Jin, M. (2020a). A serological survey of SARS-CoV-2 in cat in Wuhan. *Emerging Microbes & Infections*, *9*(1), 2013–2019.

Zhang, J.-J., Dong, X., Cao, Y.-Y., Yuan, Y.-D., Yang, Y. B., Yan, Y.-Q., Akdis, C. A., & Gao, Y.-D. (2020b). Clinical characteristics of 140 patients infected with SARS-CoV-2 in Wuhan, China. *Allergy*, *75*(7), 1730–1741.

Epilogue

Deborah Lupton

Reading through the fascinating chapters in this book, I was struck by how accounts of one nation's experience of the COVID-19 pandemic resonate with how this crisis has been experienced in similar wealthy countries across the globe. Many themes across the volume are to be found in previous investigations of COVID life undertaken by social researchers in their own countries. One example is that Danish older people and those living with disabilities reported less change in their everyday lives and routines compared with social groups who were unused to the confinement imposed by social isolation, discrimination, and marginalisation. Another example is the differences between younger people and older people evident in the research reported in this book. Young people in most countries have experienced far greater disruption to their life expectations, rites of passage, and opportunities than those who have already left the workforce and are living quiet retired lives. So too, in Denmark and across the world, people in occupations where they could not easily avoid contact with others (such as healthcare, factory, slaughterhouse, delivery and supermarket workers) were exposed to far higher levels of risk than those who could work from home. Furthermore, discussions of the policies and politics of public health measures such as lockdowns, mandated vaccines, and mass mask wearing in the Danish context repeat many of the controversies and manufactured uncertainties that have existed in other geographical regions.

As the analyses in the book's chapters demonstrate, therefore, within a single country, sociodemographic and spatial factors can play a major role in shaping COVID experiences. However, national differences are also important to consider. There are inevitably aspects of the Danish experience that are unique compared with those of citizens in other nations, even in the same region. Across this volume, the implications of the COVID crisis for the welfare state are highlighted. Here, the Danish state (along with other Nordic nations) is perhaps the most distinctive in terms of its strong public healthcare system and other social welfare support offered to its citizens. Nations where healthcare has become increasingly privatised or underfunded can offer nowhere near the benefits of the universal free healthcare that Denmark provides its citizens. Yet, as the contributions collected here demonstrate, even Denmark's superior welfare and health systems, and its ability to offer abundant vaccines and the latest therapies to citizens who contracted COVID, still confronted major challenges in managing the impacts of the pandemic. Like many other nations in the Global North, Denmark faced a rolling pattern of peaks and troughs in COVID deaths as successive waves of the disease passed through the country from January 2020.

Since the emergence of the novel coronavirus SARS-CoV-2, governments and their citizens have learnt the hard way just how unpredictable this virus is: it constantly changes in time and space as it mutates and public health responses wax and wane. Another theme across several of these chapters is the more-than-human entanglements of COVID risks. SARS-CoV-2 is a forceful agent (having already caused millions of deaths across the world) but it is only powerful when it is part of human-nonhuman assemblages, such as human bodies and their immune systems, vaccines, agents such as air purifiers, ventilation systems and face masks that prevent the virus from entering the human body. Further, other animal hosts capable of harbouring the virus, medical therapies, border closures, immigration regulations, quarantine and self-isolating facilities, public health campaigns, press conferences, case reports, news stories, and many more agents are also part of these assemblages. In certain COVID risk assemblage combinations, the potential for the virus to infect the human body and cause severe disease or death is increased, while in others, the virus is rendered impotent. The conditions in which these assemblages come together and come apart are continually changing, with the virus itself mutating as it moves from body to body and creating further complexities for pandemic management and containment.

As this pandemic continues to unfold, there are lessons to be learned globally in forensically identifying how this emergency has been confronted by diverse medical and public health systems within specific geographical locations and with a wide array of ideologies embodied in governments' approaches to COVID management. Successes and failures alike must be examined and analysed for what can help us going forward into an uncertain future, in which it has become increasingly evident exactly how political the crisis has become. A range of actors actively engage in COVID denial or minimising, working to ensure that profits of wealthy corporations and 'the economy' are privileged at the expense of effective public health measures. These include politicians, 'tame' scientists, public health and medical researchers at prestigious universities, members of think tanks, lobby groups and advisory groups. They have drawn on the playbook that has proved so successful for climate science deniers. A great silence has descended in governments and the mainstream news media worldwide on the continuing threat posed by COVID. Collections such as this book, focusing on how a single nation has adapted to the mutable virus (or failed to adapt), as well as those that can compare experiences across the globe are vitally important, particularly from the neglected Global East and Global South, which have yet to receive adequate attention in the socio-spatial analysis of this terrible, unrelenting global catastrophe.

Author biographies

Almlund, Pernille, PhD, associate professor in communication at the Department of Communication and Art, Roskilde University, Denmark. She is head of the research group Public Communication and has in her research focus on risk communication, climate communication, health communication, and political communication. She has recently contributed with a co-authored chapter to an edited volume titled *Communicating a Pandemic: Crisis Management and COVID-19 in the Nordic Countries* published by Nordicom, University of Gothenburg. The chapter is about Nordic public campaigns during COVID-19 and is titled 'Expressions of Governance, Risk, and Responsibility: Public Campaigns in the Crisis and Risk Management of COVID-19 in Denmark, Norway, and Sweden'. ORCID: orcid.org/0000-0002-0100-771X

Bech, Christine Flagstad, MSc in pharmacy, PhD student at Roskilde University/Region Zealand Hospital Pharmacy, Denmark. In her research, she combines a participatory design approach with her background as a pharmacist to facilitate task reallocation from doctors to clinical pharmacists using local configuration of the electronic health record. Other areas of interest include rational pharmacotherapy and quality improvement projects within healthcare. ORCID: orcid.org/0000-0001-6493-5452

Blaakilde, Anne Leonora, PhD, associate professor at Roskilde University, Department of People and Technology. With a background in Folklore and Ethnology from the University of Copenhagen, Blaakilde works with qualitative research, applying narrativity, discourse analyses and everyday life perspectives. Her expertise is within cultural and social gerontology; studying ageing from a cultural and social perspective, and she has researched on family life, generations, gender, migration, media and life in institutional settings. ORCID: orcid.org/0000-0002-4243-3109

Christensen, Karen, Dr.Polit., professor in health and society at the Department of People and Technology, Roskilde University, Denmark. She currently holds a Professor II position at the Faculty of Social and Health Sciences, Innland University of Applied Sciences, Lillehammer, Norway. She has researched and published in areas such as welfare state changes, comparative social policies, gendered care work, and migratory ageing. Among her publications, she has co-edited *The Routledge Handbook of Social Care Work Around the World*, 2018. ORCID orcid.org/0000-0003-0145-1957

Eilersen, Andreas Thomas, PhD, postdoc in theoretical disease modelling at the PandemiX Center at Roskilde University. His main research interests include population dynamics and mathematical and numerical modelling of epidemics. In particular, his current work focuses on the application of epidemic models in the study of historical epidemics, with a focus on smallpox and cholera in 18th- and 19th-century Denmark. ORCID: orcid.org/0000-0003-1451-7564

Falster, Emil, PhD, is a postdoctoral researcher at the Universal Design Hub/Bevica Foundation and the Department of Sociology and Social Work at Aalborg University. His research focuses on disabled children and young people and their everyday lives, as well as the Danish concept of disability and how it generates opportunities and limitations for the fulfilment of the UN Sustainable Development Goals and the Leave No One Behind agenda. ORCID: orcid.org/0000-0002-0668-0700

Gyldenkærne, Christopher, H., cand.it, PhD fellow at the Department of People and Technology, Roskilde University. In his research, Gyldenkærne specializes in applied AI and case studies of large- and small-scale healthcare technologies. He has a diverse research background and uses a range of methods, including quantitative, qualitative, and design approaches to explore the implications of implementing cutting-edge technology in healthcare. His interests lie in investigating the impact of future technologies on healthcare workers and patients. Through his research, Christopher seeks to advance our understanding of the potential of emerging technologies to transform healthcare and improve patient outcomes. ORCID: orcid.org/0000-0003-2858-7328

Holm, Jesper, associate professor, is a researcher and lecturer at the Department of People and Technology, Roskilde University. He has participated in several international research project and networks on environment, STS and transition. His main interest lies in sustainable transition approaches in various areas, environmental health, and the role of the state. Holm has previously published the book: Holm, J., Søndergaard, B., Stauning, I., & Jensen, J. O. (Eds.). (2014). *Sustainable Transition of Housing and Construction*. Frederiksberg: Frydenlund Academic. ORCID: orcid.org/0000-0003-4538-8814

Jelsøe, Erling, associate professor at the Department of People and Technology, Roskilde University. He is also affiliated with the Center for Research in Health Promotion. In his research, Jelsøe engages with a wide array of topics related to sustainable development and health aspects within agriculture and food production. This includes strategies for change within the food sector, public participation in sustainable development, introduction of new biotechnologies, and the development of health and welfare technologies and consequences for users and patients. ORCID: orcid.org/0009-0004-8262-7137

Jha, Aruna, PhD, licensed clinical social worker, assistant professor in the Social Work Department, University of Wisconsin-Whitewater, USA. Jha teaches social work practice, and advanced clinical skills courses. She uses mixed methods to research risk and protective factors for depression and suicide in immigrant populations with an emphasis on the role of cultural conflict, acculturation attitudes, and life transitions as risk factors for suicide among South Asian Americans. Dr. Jha is an international expert on suicide and presents workshops highlighting the impact of cultural values on suicidal ideation and behaviour. ORCID: orcid.org/0000-0003-0591-0997

Krogfelt, Karen A., PhD, is a professor (MSO), at the Department of Science and Environment, section of Molecular and Medical Biology, Roskilde University. Her main focus is on infectious bacteriology, in particular host-bacteria interactions, bacterial virulence, antibiotic resistance, animal models, gastrointestinal infections, diagnostics of bacterial infections. Krogfelt teaches within medical microbiology and is co-applicant in the PandemiX Center, founded by the Danish National Research Foundation 2023–2029. ORCID: orcid.org/0000-0001-7536-3453

Lehn, Sine, PhD, is an associate professor in critical health studies, Department of People and Technology, Roskilde University. Lehn is head of PhD programme Health and Society. Lehn's field of research is work and education of health professions with special focus on interprofessional collaboration, professional identities, changing conditions of work and learning. ORCID: orcid.org/0000-0002-2566-8766

Liveng, Anne, PhD, is an associate professor at the Department of People and Technology, Roskilde University. Her research interests focus on elder care, ageing, health promotion, and learning. Theoretically, she is inspired by care theories, care ethics, psychosocial theory, and critical theory. Anne as well has an interest in the development of qualitative methods and analysis, for instance, the use of arts, psychosocial methods, and other methods stemming from the humanities. She is a co-founder of the CareSam® Network (https://caresam.mau.se/) and a member of the conference committee in Nordic Health Promotion Research Network (https://nhprn.com/). ORCID: orcid.org/ 0000-0001-5920-3492

Lupton, Deborah, PhD, is a SHARP professor in the Centre for Social Research in Health and the Social Policy Research Centre and leader of the Vitalities Lab. Lupton is also the UNSW node leader, health focus area leader, and people co-leader of the Australian Research Council Centre of

Excellence for Automated Decision-Making and Society. She has a background in sociology and media and cultural studies, and her research combines qualitative and innovative social research methods with sociocultural theory. Deborah is the author/co-author of 20 books and editor/co-editor of a further ten book collections, as well as over 240 book chapters and articles. She blogs at This Sociological Life. ORCID: orcid.org/0000-0003-2658-4430

Malik, Aisha, MSc, is a data analyst at Statens Serum Institut (SSI), Denmark. Malik's work is specialized in working with healthcare organizations and technology to identify, implement, and optimize technology solutions that improve patient care, increase efficiency, and reduce costs. At SSI, she is responsible for collecting and organizing large sets of complex data from various sources. She uses this data to create visualizations and reports that effectively communicate insights to key stakeholders. In her role, Aisha ensures that the organization complies with various regulations, including policies, standards, laws, and transparency requirements. ORCID: orcid.org/0009-0001-2408-2579

Mirsepasi-Lauridsen, Hengameh Chloé, PhD, is a research scientist at the Department of Clinical Microbiology & Department of Gastroenterology, Hvidovre Hospital, Denmark and Department of Science and Environment, Section of Molecular and Medical Biology, Roskilde University. She has decades of experience as a clinical and molecular microbiologist. Specialized in gastrointestinal diseases and microbiology. Inventor of faecal microbiota transplantation capsule used to cure antibiotic resistance to *Clostridioides difficile* infection, etc. Mirsepasi-Lauridsen is the inventor of innovative faecal virus transplantation capsules in collaboration with Copenhagen University. ORCID: orcid.org/0000-0002-5883-3262

Mønsted, Troels, PhD, is an associate professor in digitalization of healthcare at the Department of Informatics, University of Oslo. He is a member of the board of the Danish Society for Digital Health and is affiliated to the HISP Centre (Health Information Systems Program), Oslo. In his research, he combines qualitative methods and action research in investigating design and use of patient-centred technologies and information infrastructures in healthcare. ORCID: orcid.org/0000-0002-5807-0285

Poder, Søren Kølholt, MSc, is PhD student at the PandemiX Center, Roskilde University. In his current research, Poder is engaging with a historical-epidemiological perspective on smallpox. He has previously conducted research on the possible significance of the structural features of historical socio-economics networks in terms of the spatial diffusion and local impact of the 1918 influenza. Methodically, Poder has developed a field within historical research that integrates digital humanities and extensive datasets based on the methodical use of crowdsourcing and collective intelligence.

Rendtorff, Jacob Dahl, PhD, and Dr. Scient. Adm., is a professor of philosophy and ethics at Roskilde University. Rendtorff's research has a broad perspective on bioethics and biolaw, philosophy of management, business ethics, sustainability, corporate social responsibility, human rights, political theory, and philosophy of law. Rendtorff is editor-in-chief of the *International Journal of Ethics and Systems*, Emerald. Recent publications are *Biolaw, Economics and Sustainable Governance: Addressing the Challenges of a Post-Pandemic World*, Routledge 2022 (together with Erick Waldés) and *Philosophy of Management and Sustainability. Rethinking Business Ethics and Corporate Social Responsibility in Sustainable Development*, Emerald 2019. Rendtorff's main research interests are bioethics and biolaw, sustainability and cosmopolitan business ethics. Rendtorff is president of European Business Ethics Network (EBEN) and member of the Steering Committee of FISP (International Federation of Philosophical Societies). ORCID: orcid.org/0000-0001-9021-4720

Runciman, Christina Naike, MA in psychology and pedagogy & educational studies, is external lecturer at the Department of People and Technology, Roskilde University and a professional support teacher for students at Roskilde University and Copenhagen University.

Runciman's research interests are in particular related to couples living apart together (LATT) and deals with areas of intimacy and distance, ethically mixed couples and decolonization as well as student performance in higher education. ORCID: orcid.org/0009-0003-7204-9938

Simonsen, Jesper, PhD, is a professor of participatory design at the Department of People and Technology, Roskilde University, Denmark. He has since 1991 conducted participatory design research in collaboration with industry, since 2005 specifically within the healthcare sector. His research is focused on how information technology designers can cooperate with users and their management especially when relating to the clarification of goals, formulation of needs, and designing, implementing, realizing, and evaluating coherent visions for change. Co-author of *Routledge International Handbook of Participatory Design* (Routledge, 2012) and *Design Research: Synergies from Interdisciplinary Perspectives* (Routledge, 2010). ORCID: orcid.org/0000-0002-1864-7158

Simonsen, Lone, PhD, is a professor of population health sciences/epidemiology at Roskilde University, Denmark, and director of PandemiX – a Center of Excellence. Through approximately 30 years of research experience and previous positions at CDC, WHO, NIH, George Washington University and Copenhagen University, Simonsen's research has covered COVID-19, pandemic influenza, RSV, HIV/AIDS, tuberculosis, SARS, big data modelling, disease surveillance, smallpox, and vaccine programme evaluation. She pioneered novel areas of study, including historical epidemiology, and managed to challenge a few public health paradigms over the years. During COVID-19, she advised Danish health authorities and government and was widely cited in national and international media. ORCID: orcid.org/0000-0003-1535-8526

Singla, Ms. Rashmi, PhD, is an associate professor, Department of People and Technology, Roskilde University. She is also affiliated to NGO –TTT (Transcultural Therapeutic Team for Ethnic Minority Youth/Families). Singla is engaged in teaching, research, international projects, and publication within social psychological/interdisciplinary frameworks. Her focus is on dynamics related to movements across borders, especially migration, transnationalism, decolonization, family/couple relationships, global health, and psychosocial intervention. She is advisor for Society Intercultural Psychology Denmark and *Learning Curve* Journal India as well as a board member of Nordic Migration Research and expert reviewer for the European Science Foundation. ORCID: orcid.org/0000-0002-7981-1169

Sørensen, Camilla Adler, MSc, is a research scientist at the Department of Science and Environment, Section of Molecular and Medical Biology, Roskilde University. Her expertise is within microbiology, in particular host-bacteria interactions, bacterial virulence. The main focus is on developing diagnostic methods for infectious diseases by serological and molecular methods. ORCID: orcid.org/0009-0009-1978-200X

Sørensen, Pelle Korsbæk, PhD, is a lecturer in nursing at the Research & Development Unit at University College Absalon, Denmark. He is the former chairperson of the Nordic Sociological Association (2016–2018). He makes use of different methodological approaches, and he teaches in research design and mixed methods. His interest is in sociology of health and his main areas of research is moral and ethical distress and psychosocial working environment among health professionals. ORCID: orcid.org/0000-0003-1813-5344

Thualagant, Nicole, PhD, is an associate professor and head of Study in Critical Health Studies at the University of Roskilde. She is also a member of the scientific committee in the Nordic Health Promotion Research Network meeting twice a year at WHO in Copenhagen. As a sociologist, her interest is in health policies, more especially how health policies interfere with more intimate spheres of social life in contemporary welfare societies. ORCID: orcid.org/0000-0002-5197-8979

Troelsen, Jesper T., PhD, is a professor and head of the molecular and medical biology section. Department of Science and Environment, Section of Molecular and Medical Biology, Roskilde University. A main research focus is an investigation of the relationship between intestinal function, genes, and disease, and the identification of biomarkers. Our research aims to understand how genetic factors impact the functioning of the intestines, and to develop new ways to diagnose and treat various diseases. ORCID: orcid.org/0000-0002-4177-3267

Vagtholm, Isabella, PhD student in the Department of Social Sciences and Business at Roskilde University. Her research centres on how social categories, including gender, age, class, ethnicity, race, and (dis)ability, affect the subjectification of children and young people. This entails a focus on the construction of norms, power dynamics, and a particular emphasis on everyday life perspectives. She has contributed to the field of norm-critical pedagogy by advocating for the significance of incorporating (dis)ability as an integral dimension of an intersectional approach. ORCID: orcid.org/0009-0006-0459-774X

van Wijhe, Maarten, PhD, assistant professor in statistical epidemiology at the PandemiX Center, Department of Science and Environment, Roskilde University. He teaches statistics and epidemiology and uses a broad range of approaches in his research. His interests are in historical epidemics and pandemics, the impact of vaccinations and other mitigation strategies, as well as the use of health registers for research. He has a special interest in merging qualitative historical research with quantitative methods. ORCID: orcid.org/0000-0001-9216-8393

Warming, Hanne, PhD, is professor of sociology and childhood, and head of the research group 'Social Dynamics and Change' at Roskilde University. Her research fields of expertise include childhood and youth, everyday life, Children's lived citizenship and citizenship learning, methodology and ethics in childhood and youth research, and how childhood and youth research can contribute to the wider scholarly fields. Recent publications include *Society and Social Change through the Prism of Childhood*, special issue of Children's Geographies (2022), and *Lived Citizenship on the Edge of Society: Rights, Belonging, Intimate Life and Spatiality*, Palgrave Macmillan (2017). ORCID: orcid.org/0000-0003-2212-8876

Index

Note: **Bold** page numbers refer to tables and *italic* page numbers refer to figures.

For Product Safety Concerns and Information please contact our
EU representative GPSR@taylorandfrancis.com Taylor & Francis
Verlag GmbH, Kaufingerstraße 24, 80331 München, Germany